T0303908

Alcohol and Substance Abuse in Women and Children

The *Advances in Alcohol & Substance Abuse* series:

Alcohol and Substance Abuse in Women and Children

Barry Stimmel, MD
Editor

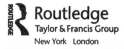

Routledge
Taylor & Francis Group
New York   London

Routledge is an imprint of the
Taylor & Francis Group, an informa business

Alcohol and Substance Abuse in Women and Children has also been published as *Advances in Alcohol & Substance Abuse*, Volume 5, Number 3, Spring 1986.

Reprinted 2009 by Routledge

Library of Congress Cataloging-in-Publication Data
Main entry under title:

Alcohol and substance abuse in women and children.

Also published as Advances in alcohol & substance abuse, v. 5, no 3, spring 1986.
Bibliography: p.
1. Alcoholism—Psychological aspects. 2. Substance abuse—Psychological aspects.
3. Women—Alcohol use. 4. Women—Drug use. 5 Children—Alcohol use.
6. Children—Drug use. 7. Family psychotherapy. I Stimmel, Barry, 1939-   .
[DNLM: 1. Alcoholism—in infancy & childhood. 2. Alcoholism—psychology.
3. Substance Abuse—in infancy & childhood. 4. Substance Abuse—psychology.
5. Women—psychology.
W1 AS432 v.5 no.3 / WM 270 A3557]
RC565.A393 1986   616.86   86-251
ISBN 0-86656-575-2

Alcohol and Substance Abuse in Women and Children

Advances in Alcohol & Substance Abuse
Volume 5, Number 3

CONTENTS

Alcohol and Substance Abuse in Women and Children

EDITORIAL

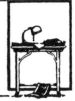

Factors Associated
With Alcohol and Substance Abuse
in Women and Children

Although substance abuse in adolescents has always been of considerable concern, until recently the abuse of drugs by women and younger children has been somewhat neglected. Surveys of the use of psychotropic drugs have consistently documented proportionately more women to use both prescription and illicit, nonopiate drugs than men, with the use of psychotropes by women almost twice that of men for each class of drugs as well as for any given agent.[1,2] Unlike drug use, alcohol abuse by women has been a matter of concern for more than a decade. Since the 1970s, the prevalence of women's drinking has remained fairly stable. Recent data by Wilsnack et al. suggest that, in general, women remain predominantly light drinkers, with abstinence common over the age of 50 and heavy drinking most often seen between the ages of 35 and 49.[3]

Hypotheses abound to explain current alcohol and substance abuse in women and children. These include the increasing stress placed on women to compete in the marketplace, the lack of parental supervision due to the economic

1

necessity of two wage earners in the family, and the general "permissive" nature of our society condoning experimentation with substances viewed as harmless, such as marijuana.[2,4] The factors related to alcohol and substance abuse in women and children and the role of the family unit in fostering their use have been infrequently assessed. This issue of Advances focuses on substance abuse in women and children, with particular emphasis on the modifying role played by the family unit.

The demographics of alcohol use by women have been studied by Wilsnack et al.[3] In general, women at the lowest economic and educational strata drink less than others, with 9% with college degrees and 15% with household incomes of $50,000 or more drinking heavily as compared to a 6% overall prevalence of heavy drinking. Religion was an important factor in decreasing drinking patterns, with heavier drinking most common among women with no religious preference. Ethnicity was also related to drinking patterns, with 45% of black women abstaining compared to 38% of white women.

Of particular interest was the role of the family in women's drinking patterns. Women who had never married were found to drink at a significantly higher level between the ages of 21 and 34. Among single women working full-time, 49% were moderate to heavy drinkers—more than twice that seen among married women. Women in a common-law relationship drank significantly more than women who were married, with none of these women abstainers and 20% heavy drinkers. These findings suggest that a stable family relationship within the confines of marriage appears to be associated with decreasing alcohol consumption.

This is not true, however, with respect to the prevalence of drinking problems in women who are married to drinking spouses. For each level of spouse consumption of alcohol, women were found to drink in a manner similar to their husbands, with the exception of wives of husbands who were clearly problem drinkers. These women, perhaps aware of the hazards of excessive alcohol consumption, were significantly less likely to consume alcohol than wives of frequent drinkers.

In this issue of Advances, Wilsnack et al. extend their study in an attempt to relate negative life experiences to patterns of alcohol consumption.[5] Of their stratified sample of 917 women, weighted to include a cohort of 500 moderate to heavy drinkers, 24% of all women had a depressive episode of two weeks or more in duration, 23% were regular users of tranquilizers, 7% were users of marijuana and between 7% and 28% had adverse reproductive experiences, ranging from infertility to births of infants with severe defects. In studying the relationships of these adverse events to drinking patterns, it appeared that these traumatic events usually occurred prior to the onset of heavy drinking. The hazards of alcohol consumption in one prone to depressive episodes are emphasized by their findings of suicide attempts in 25% of women drinking more than twenty-four drinks per week as compared to 3% of women drinking less than this amount. Severe, depressive reactions were seen in 53% as compared to 10% of the light drinkers. These data suggest that, in those women susceptible to alcohol abuse, adverse life experiences will result in an increase in alcohol consumption. However, it appears unlikely that women will become drinkers in middle or old age if drinking patterns were nonexistent in their youth.

The use of illicit drugs, nonmedical use of prescription drugs and medical use of psychoactive substances by women, as demonstrated by Kaestner et al. in this issue, continue to increase.[6] These investigators document a dramatic increase of use in women between the ages of 18 and 34, with the use of medically prescribed psychoactive substances seen in 30% of married women as compared to men. Similar to alcohol use, single women employed full time have considerably higher rates of use of both illicit substances and prescription drugs when compared to housewives. This increase in use by women in the marketplace compared to housewives may vary between twofold to more than fivefold, depending on the specific group of drugs. This is most dramatically demonstrated by Mittleman and Wetli in a review of deaths associated with recreational cocaine use.[7] These authors noted that whereas prior to 1978 the typical cocaine overdose occurred in a 26-year old Caucasian male, at present, the average age has increased to 29 years, with 42% women.

Since a strong family unit appears to discourage substance abuse, it would be expected that family therapy would be helpful in attempting to rehabilitate the substance abuser. Several studies involving substance abuse have indeed demonstrated the effectiveness of family therapy in supporting the abstinent state even when only one family member was consistently involved in therapy.[8] This latter finding is particularly helpful as, not infrequently, many members of a family unit are either unable or unwilling to engage in therapy. In this issue Kosten et al., through a pilot project involving eight addicts and their families, systematically compare family functioning before and after family therapy.[9] A significant improvement at the conclusion of therapy is demonstrated, with only one of the eight patients relapsing during a ten-month follow-up. Although these results are quite encouraging, clearly further controlled studies are in order to determine the benefits that may be obtained from family therapy in narcotic dependence.

The use of alcohol and other drugs by the young remains a matter of concern. A recent study by Johnston et al. provides some cause for satisfaction.[10] Based on samplings from 125 to 140 public and private high schools across the country, it appears that the decline in overall illicit drug use, which began in the early 1980s, continues, with the prevalence of adolescents reporting drug use dropping from 54% to 49%. Most impressive is the decline in marijuana use from 37% in 1979 to 27% in 1983. Amphetamines, methaqualone, LSD, barbiturates, tranquilizers and also PCP have similarly continued to decline. However, the use of inhalers, heroin and other opiates remains unchanged. Cocaine use appears to have leveled off after more than doubling between 1975 and 1979, with a current prevalence of 11%. However, those in the field have noted a dramatic increase in cocaine use among adults. In addition, in specific areas of the nation, notably the cities, drug use by children remains considerable. There is, therefore, little cause for complacency.

With respect to alcohol and tobacco use, although indicators do not document an increased consumption, their use is considerable. By the end of the senior year in high school, nearly 93% of students have tried alcohol, with 69% having drank in the preceding month and 11% having consumed five or more consecutive drinks at least once in the preceding week. Overall drug use in high school remains considerable. Nearly two-thirds of students have used an illicit drug before they finish high school, with 40% using drugs other than marijuana.

Daily smoking occurred in 20% of the students, with 31% having smoked in the preceding month. Lest one think that smoking should be viewed as neither an addictive nor an abusing substance, it is important to emphasize that nicotine is indeed addicting, with dependency most often beginning in adolescence.[11,12] In fact, smoking is responsible for more deaths annually than alcohol and drug abuse combined. It is the single largest preventable cause of disease and death in this country.[13]

Although one might assume that with increasing education and maturity among an upwardly mobile population drug abuse would decrease, recent findings by Friend and Koushki demonstrate that this might not be true.[14] In a study of 459 college students, 81% of entering freshmen drank and 34% used drugs. After remaining in college for a year, approximately 16% of male abstainers began to drink and 18% to use drugs (p. < 0.01). These rates remained stable throughout the remainder of college. Women showed a similar pattern with respect to alcohol; however, they did experience a subsequent rise in drug use.

Much greater efforts are needed to determine the factors responsible for children initiating drug use, as well as implementing measures that will be effective in diminishing this use. Factors that one would predict to be related to such use include ethnicity, family constellation, availability and gender. Maddahian et al. in this issue review the relationships between ethnicity, income and availability and substance abuse in adolescents.[15] These authors convincingly demonstrate consistent, significant differences in patterns and types of substances abused by ethnicity. Income, also an important predictor, loses its predictive value when availability increases. These observations are of critical importance in developing treatment strategies emphasizing the importance of community-based treatment programs.

Oei et al. in this issue review factors associated with the initiation of smoking in nine year olds.[16] Of the 800 children surveyed, 30% had tried smoking at some time. Smokers were more likely to have: (1) both parents smoke; (2) friends who smoked; (3) also tried alcohol; (4) developed behavioral or emotional problems; and (5) performed less well at school. For reasons which remain less than clear, a significant association between the home environment and a tendency to have tried smoking and other drugs could not be documented. This is in contrast to the findings of Beecher concerning "dictated deviance" and drug use.[17] Beecher hypothesized that substance abuse could be traced directly back to the message transmitted in the home environment.

It is interesting that Kaestner et al. have found a difference in behavioral problems between boys and girls in the presence of similar rates of substance abuse.[6] Girls appear to develop behavioral problems at a much lower rate than boys. Whether this is due to girls having more "discreet" behavioral problems or to bias on the part of observers, resulting in less detection, is unclear. These findings, however, warrant further study.

In this issue Brook et al. review risk factors associated with alcohol consumption in over 900 adolescents.[18] These investigators noted a marked protective effect of a stable family unit. Protective personality attributes also served as buffers to alcohol consumption, as did high achievement. Positive parent-child relationships, lack of drug models, identification with the mother and a strong positive relationship with the father all tended to diminish the risk of drinking. Contrarily, maternal nonidentification and oversolicitiousness of both parents were associated with both drug and alcohol use.

Heroin dependency, always a matter of special concern in the cities, is addressed by Brunswick and Messeri in a study of urban black youths between the ages of 18 and 23.[19] Among the more interesting findings are the differential effects of treatment between men and women. Men entering treatment were found to have only marginally benefited whereas women demonstrated markedly beneficial effects. For each year of use prior to entering treatment, a woman's probability of abstinence was lower than that of a man's. However, after the therapeutic experience, the annual probability for a woman to remain abstinent was comparatively enhanced and, when expressed absolutely, was even greater than the probability of post-treatment abstinence for men. The odds that a woman heroin user would abstain each year following treatment increased more than sixfold over that of an untreated woman. Sample size did not allow conclusions to be drawn as to the reason for these differences.

The papers in this issue document the prevalence of alcohol

and substance abuse among women and children, as well as the importance of the family unit in discouraging and even preventing such use. Of most concern in addressing this issue is the early identification of a potential abuse problem. It is therefore incumbent on physicians engaged in primary care, as well as other health professionals, to become comfortable in identifying those at risk to provide intervention as early as possible.

It is important to emphasize that the occurrence of even a single episode of acute intoxication in adolescence may herald the presence of a significant problem. Stephenson et al., in a review of 171 acutely intoxicated adolescents admitted to an emergency room, found these youngsters at a significantly higher risk for alcohol and polydrug abuse, as well as psychologic dependency, as compared to a randomly selected group from the surrounding community.[20] Success is more frequently seen if the intervention begins prior to the actual establishment of dependency. All those in the health professions must be sufficiently informed to recognize alcohol and substance abuse as early as possible.

Barry Stimmel, MD

REFERENCES

1. Parry HJ. The use of psychotropic drugs by U.S. adults. Pub Health Service Reports. 1968; 83:799–810.
2. Parry HJ, Balter MB, Mellinger GD, Cisin IH, Manheimer DI National patterns of psychotherapeutic drug use. Arch Gen Psychiat. 1973; 28:769–83.
3 Wilsnack RW, Wilsnack SC, Klassen AD. Women's drinking and drinking problems: patterns from a 1981 national survey. Am J Pub Hlth. 1984; 74:1231–8.
4. Johnson PB. Sex differences, women's roles and alcohol use: preliminary national data. J Soc Issues. 1982; 38:93–116.
5. Wilsnack RW, Klassen AD, Wilsnack SC. Retrospective analysis of lifetime changes in women's drinking behavior. Advances in Alcohol & Substance Abuse. 1986; 5(3):9–28.
6. Kaestner E, Frank B, Marel R, Schmeidler J. Substance use among females in New York State: catching up with the males. Advances in Alcohol & Substance Abuse. 1986; 5(3):29–49.
7 Mittleman RE, Wetli CV. Death caused by recreational cocaine use: an update. JAMA. 1984; 252:1889–93.
8. Study of two brief family therapy approaches. Clinical Research Notes. National Institute on Drug Abuse. June, 1984; p. 5.
9. Kosten TR, Hogan I, Jalali B, Steidl J, Kleber HD. The effect of multiple

family therapy on addict family functioning: a pilot study. Advances in Alcohol & Substance Abuse. 1986; 5(3):51–62.

10. Johnson LD, O'Malley PM, Bachman JG. Highlights from drugs and American high school students 1975–1983. U.S. Department of Health and Human Services, Alcohol, Drug Abuse and Mental Health Administration, National Institute on Drug Abuse, Rockville, Maryland. 1984.

11. Pollin W. Why people smoke cigarettes. Public Health Service Pub No. 83-50185, Rockville, Maryland.

12. Russell MAH. Tobacco smoking and nicotine dependence. In: Gibbins, RJ, Israel Y, Kalant H et al., eds. Research Advances in Alcohol and Drug Problems. New York: John Wiley & Sons, 1976: 1–47

13. Pollin W. The role of the addictive process as a key step in causation of all tobacco-related diseases. JAMA. 1984; 252:2874.

14. Friend KE, Koushki PA. Student substance use: stability and change across college years. Internat J Addict. 1984; 19:571–75.

15. Maddahian E, Newcomb MD, Bentler PM. Adolescents' substance use impact of ethnicity, income, and availability. Advances in Alcohol and Substance Abuse. 1986; 5(3):63–78.

16. Oei TPS, Egan AM, Silva PA. Factors associated with the initiation of "smoking" in nine year old children. Advances in Alcohol & Substance Abuse. 1986; 5(3):79–89.

17. Beecher EM and Editors of Consumer Reports. Licit and Illicit Drugs. Boston: Little Brown and Co., 1972:494–96.

18. Brook JS, Whiteman M, Gordon AS, Nomura C, Brook DW. Onset of adolescent drinking: a longitudinal study of intrapersonal and interpersonal antecedents. Advances in Alcohol & Substance Abuse. 1986; 5(3):91–110.

19. Brunswick AF, Messeri PA. Pathways to heroin abstinence: a longitudinal study of urban black youth. Advances in Alcohol & Substance Abuse. 1986; 5(3):111–135.

20. Stephenson JN, Moberg DP, Daniels BJ, Robertson JF. Treating the intoxicated adolescent: a need for comprehensive services. JAMA. 1984; 252:1884–7.

Retrospective Analysis of Lifetime Changes in Women's Drinking Behavior

Richard W. Wilsnack, PhD
Albert D. Klassen, MA
Sharon C. Wilsnack, PhD

ABSTRACT. Retrospective data on drinking behavior and related life experiences have been a neglected resource in research on alcohol use in the general population. Data from a 1981 national survey of women's drinking indicate the potential value of retrospective data analysis. The 1981 data provide comparative ages of onset for drinking behavior, drinking consequences, and health problems, and allow comparisons among different cohorts of women. The data also show the variability in women's lifetime drinking patterns and the time-ordering of heavy drinking in relation to onset of depression and reproductive dysfunction.

To understand the causes and consequences of alcohol abuse, better data are needed on the timing of drinking behavior in relation to other behavior and experiences, for several reasons. Drinking may be both a cause and a consequence of physical illness, depression, marital and employment problems, and other stressful life experiences; time-ordered data

Richard W. Wilsnack is Professor, and Albert D. Klassen a Senior Research Associate, with the Department of Sociology, University of North Dakota. Sharon C. Wilsnack is Professor, Department of Neuroscience, University of North Dakota School of Medicine.

This research was supported by Research Grant No. AA04610 from the National Institute on Alcohol Abuse and Alcoholism. Portions of this paper were presented at the Annual Meeting, International Society for Biomedical Research on Alcoholism and Research Society on Alcoholism, Santa Fe, New Mexico, June 24-29, 1984. We are grateful to Karen G. Knutson for assistance with computer programming. Reprint requests to Richard W. Wilsnack, Department of Sociology, University of North Dakota, Grand Forks ND 58202.

are necessary to unravel these relationships. Drinking may vary so much over time that drinking patterns at one point of time may be poor predictors of alcohol use earlier or later in life. And data on drinking histories may be essential to evaluate to what extent the influences on drinking, and the effects of drinking, may be age-specific, or time-limited, or delayed, or cumulative over time.

The most respected method for obtaining time-ordered data about drinking patterns has been multiwave longitudinal research with a panel of respondents.[1-4] However, such multiwave panel studies are expensive and therefore scarce; their timeframe is often limited to a few years; attrition of respondents can weaken or bias their samples; and they have often not tried to learn what respondents were doing or experiencing at times other than when the data were being collected. It is imperative, therefore, to augment the data that have been available from panel studies, by improving the collection of retrospective data, so that information recalled by respondents will allow analyses of time sequences, time periods, and ages of onset of drinking behavior and related lifetime experiences. Obtaining such retrospective data from cross-sectional studies could compensate for the expense, time limits, and sample attrition in panel studies. Heretofore, however, cross-sectional surveys of drinking behavior have not provided much data suitable for time-ordered analyses.

It is clearly feasible to obtain and use such data. Research has shown that it is possible to obtain retrospective data on important life events[5-9] and on past drinking behavior and drinking consequences,[10-14] including lifetime drinking patterns,[15-16] with sufficient reliability and validity for time-ordered analyses of aggregated data. Furthermore, there are methodological strategies that can reduce or compensate for errors of recall,[7,17-19] including common-sense practices of asking only about facts of events and behavior that are likely to be important and unusual in the respondent's life, and *not* asking for more details than a respondent is likely to remember. There are also sophisticated procedures available for analyzing time-sequences of life-historical data,[20-22] although these procedures have yet to be exploited for the analysis of histories of drinking behavior and drinking-related problems.

Simpler time-ordered analyses based on retrospective data

have long been a part of clinical research. Most recently, such analyses have been used to show a higher incidence of stressful life events in the lives of people who would subsequently become alcohol abusers than in the lives of matched non-abusers at the same ages,[23-25] and to show that some types of alcohol abusers (such as so-called "reactive" alcoholics) are more likely to be influenced by antecedent health problems or stressful experiences than other types of alcohol abusers (such as so-called "essential" or "primary" alcoholics).[26,27] However, there has been little comparable time-ordered analysis of retrospective data on drinking in the general population, and with few exceptions,[25,28] the clinical research has studied drinking as either a cause or a consequence of other experiences but not as both.

To indicate the potential gains from collecting retrospective data in cross-sectional surveys, we present here some preliminary analyses of such data from a large national sample of women in the general population. The data include information on lifetime drinking changes, and dates of initial experiences with a variety of major life events and behavior changes. After describing patterns of lifetime drinking as reported by women in the survey, we analyze how women's experiences with depression and with reproductive problems are related to lifetime maximum drinking levels as compared with current drinking levels. We then analyze how heavy drinking precedes and/or follows depression and adverse reproductive experiences, among women who report both heavy drinking and these experiences. These preliminary findings can serve as stimuli for more subtle and complex analyses of causes and consequences of women's drinking.

METHODS

Sample

The data presented here come from a 1981 U.S. national survey of a stratified sample of 917 women, including 500 moderate to heavy drinking women (who reported consuming at least 4 drinks a week), 378 lighter-drinking or abstaining women, and 39 self-reported former problem drinkers. Previous surveys[29,30] have indicated that women who report drinking 4 or more drinks per week represent approximately the 20% of women with the heaviest alcohol consumption. The stratification procedure involved an initial screening interview with 94% of the women in 4032 households, after which survey interviews were completed with 89% of the moderate-to-heavy drinkers and former problem drinkers, and 83% of the light drinkers and abstainers eligible for interviews (a systematic subsample of 1 in 4 of such women). All but 4 of the 120 interviewers were women, and none had a history of alcohol-related problems or moral objections to the use of alcohol. Interviews took place between September and December 1981, so as to be completed before the onset of holiday drinking. Sampling and survey fieldwork were conducted by the National Opinion Research Center. The sample excluded women who were under age 21 or living in institutional settings. For comparison purposes, a representative sample of 396 men was also interviewed, although this paper presents only the women's data.

Demographic characteristics of the 1981 sample correspond quite closely to characteristics of the general U.S. female population as reported in two sources of comparative national data: the 1980 *Statistical Abstract of the United States*[31] and the 1980 General Social Survey conducted by the National Opinion Research Center.[32] For example, for women's occupational categories (white collar, blue collar, service workers, and farm workers), the percentages in the 1981 survey did not differ significantly from those in the 1980 *Statistical Abstract,* with the exception that the 1981 survey contained fewer farm workers (0.1% vs. 1.2%). In the 1981 survey, the percentage of women who were black matched the 1980 figures (10%) and the distributions of education levels among black women did not differ significantly. However, compared with the 1980 *Statistical Abstract,* the 1981 survey contained a larger percentage of white women with at least some college education (39% vs. 28% for white women 25 and older) and a smaller percentage of white women with no high school education (11% vs. 17%).

Percentages of women in 6 of 8 age groups did not differ between the 1981 survey and the 1980 *Statistical Abstract;* exceptions were that the 1981 survey included more women aged

30-44 (33% vs. 28%) and fewer women over 75 (4% vs. 7%). Distributions of marital status were similar for 1980 and 1981 in 6 of 8 age groups; minor differences occurred in the percentages of divorced and never-married women aged 55-64, and in the percentages of widowed, married, and never-married women over age 75. Overall, the 1981 sample appears generally representative of the U.S. adult female population at the time of the survey. Additional information on the demographic characteristics of the 1981 sample, and on relationships between demographic characteristics and women's drinking behavior, is provided in R. Wilsnack, S. Wilsnack, and A. Klassen;[33] and in S. Wilsnack, R. Wilsnack, and A. Klassen.[34]

Measures

The survey questionnaire, administered in privacy, took 1½ to 2 hours to complete. The questionnaire contained detailed questions about alcohol consumption, drinking contexts, problems resulting from drinking, symptoms of alcohol dependence, and attitudes and beliefs about drinking. Other questions dealt with demographic characteristics, family history, self-concept, role performances, stressful life experiences, social support, symptoms of anxiety and depression, physical health (including obstetrical and gynecological problems), sexual experience, use of drugs other than alcohol, and participation in antisocial behavior.

Data on lifetime changes in drinking were obtained by a procedure adapted from Robins.[35] Each respondent who was more than a minimal drinker (more than one drink a month in the preceding year), or who reported ever having wanted to reduce or stop drinking, was asked at what age she began drinking. She was also asked how much she typically drank at that time in terms of specified categories of frequency and drinks per occasion. Then she was asked at what ages (if ever) the pattern of drinking changed, and how it changed in terms of the quantity and frequency categories. A respondent could report up to six different stages of drinking history, but only 2% reported as many as five stages.

To analyze levels and changes of alcohol consumption in drinking histories, we estimated the number of drinks per day consumed by women reporting each possible combination of drinking frequency (drinking days per week) and drinking quantity (number of drinks per drinking day). The drinking histories had three categories of drinking frequency (less than 1 day per week, 1–3 days per week, 4 or more days per week) and three categories of drinking quantity (1–3 drinks per day, 4–5 drinks per day, 6 or more drinks per day). Thus there were nine possible combinations of drinking frequency and quantity. Each quantity-frequency combination allowed a certain range of average daily consumption in drinks per day. Our estimate of drinks per day for each quantity-frequency combination was the *median* number of drinks per day *currently* consumed by women whose current drinking was within the possible range of average daily consumption for that quantity and frequency. We used medians rather than mean drinks per day or range midpoints because the distributions of women's drinks per day were skewed, with more cases at the lower ends of distributions. The estimated drinks per day for the nine combinations of drinking frequency and quantity are given in Table 1.

Elsewhere in the interview, respondents also reported their ages at their first and most recent experiences of various reproductive problems, and their first and most recent experiences of two-week or longer periods of multiple depressive symptoms. Questions about obstetrical and gynecological problems were adapted from several health screening inventories.[36,37] Depression questions were from the NIMH Diagnostic Interview Schedule (DIS).[38] Criteria for a depressive

Table 1. Assigned Values of Drinks per Day for Categories of Drinking Quantity and Frequency in Questions about Stages of Drinking History

	Quantity		
Frequency	1-3 Drinks/Day	4-5 Drinks/Day	6 or More Drinks/Day
Less Than 1 Day per Week	.07	.43	.57
1-3 Days per Week	.29	1.07	1.68
4 or More Days per Week	1.50	2.86	5.93

episode included (1) a period of depressed mood lasting two or more weeks, accompanied by (2) three or more depressive symptoms, including sleep and appetite disturbances, fatigue, psychomotor retardation or agitation, loss of sexual interest, feelings of worthlessness, cognitive changes, and suicidal thoughts or behavior. Earlier analyses of the 1981 survey data have found relationships between high levels of current alcohol consumption and increased lifetime rates of various obstetrical and gynecological disorders[39] and between current alcohol consumption and lifetime rates of depressive symptoms, depressive episodes, and suicidal behavior.[33]

Data Analysis

To compensate for unequal probabilities of respondent selection, so that the data would represent the general population as closely as possible, each case was weighted by the product of 5 weighting variables. The weighting variables compensated for variations in (1) probabilities of household selection, (2) nonresponse rates for screening interviews (by segment), (3) nonresponse rates for the survey questionnaire (by segment), (4) missing dwelling units at sampled household addresses, and (5) stratification by gender and drinking level. Stratification required a weighting of 4.0 for responses of light-drinking or abstaining women, who had been subsampled on a 1 out of 4 basis.

Calculations of the percentages and measures of association reported in this paper involved weighted cases, enabling us to estimate what the patterns of drinking changes and their timing relative to other life events would be in the general female population. Tables show both weighted and unweighted cases for each comparison. Additional details of the sampling frame and weighting procedures are given in R. Wilsnack et al.[33]

RESULTS

Utility and Reliability of Drinking Histories

Among women who had been more than minimal drinkers in the preceding year (having more than one drink a month on the average), 94% provided complete information about their levels of alcohol consumption at all the stages of their drinking histories. Of the women who provided these complete drinking histories, 99.6% also reported their ages at the onset and all subsequent changes of their drinking. Of the 1592 reported lifetime changes in drinking patterns, there was only one instance of a reversal of ages for two consecutive stages of drinking, and only one instance of a drinking change reported at an age older than the respondent claimed to be.

Over 90% of the women who provided information on their drinking histories indicated that their last reported level of drinking was also their current level of drinking. For these women we had an independent measure of current drinking levels from detailed questions elsewhere about beer, wine, and liquor consumed in the preceding 30 days. Ten values of current drinking levels derived from the lifetime drinking histories for these women correlated .63 with a continuous-variable measure of current drinking from the detailed questions about recent beer, wine, and liquor consumption. Where differences occurred between the two measures, the more detailed questions about recent consumption of specific beverages tended to produce higher estimates of drinking levels (see also Williams, Aitken, & Malin).[40]

Health-Related Experiences: Prevalence and Timing

Women had little difficulty recalling ages when a variety of health-related life experiences first occurred. Table 2 summarizes data on the prevalence of seven such experiences and the median ages of first occurrence. Ninety-eight percent of the women answered the questions about these experiences, and 93% or more of the women reporting these experiences were able to give the ages of first occurrence.

The patterns in Table 2 are rather unsurprising, which may add to the credibility of the retrospective reports. The weighted data indicate that the median ages for first experiencing the four reproductive problems were in the mid-20's. Miscarriage or stillbirth was the most common such experience, reported by 28% of the women who had ever been pregnant. Regular use of marijuana was rarely reported and was likely to have developed by late adolescence, but 23% of all women reported regular use of tranquilizers at some time, beginning this use at a median age

Table 2. Percentages of Women with Various Life Experiences and Median Age
of First Experience[a]

Life Experience	Percent With Experience	Median Age of First Experience
Depressive Episode[b]	24%	27
Regular Use of Tranquilizers	23%	37
Regular Use of Marijuana	7%	18
Infertility for At Least One Year	13%	24
Among Women Ever Pregnant		
Miscarriage or Stillbirth	28%	25
Premature Delivery	11%	25
Baby with Birth Defects	7%	25

[a]Percentages are based on weighted data. The first four items apply to
all women, unweighted N=917, weighted N=2552. The last three items apply to
all women ever pregnant, unweighted N=720, weighted N=2080. These N's
include respondents with missing data for particular items of information.

[b]Two-week or longer period of depressed mood plus 3 or more depressive
symptoms.

of 37. One woman in four reported having experienced a depressive episode; the median age for the first episode was 27. At the time of the survey, the median age among all women respondents was 42.

Drinking Experiences: Prevalence and Timing

Only 28% of women respondents claimed that they had always abstained from alcohol. Among women who were more than minimal drinkers in the year before the survey, the median age for beginning to drink was 18, and 87% had begun drinking by age 21. One might expect the median age for onset of drinking to be higher in older age groups, which include women who have had an opportunity to start drinking later in life; however, even among women drinkers 65 and older, 72% said they had begun drinking before age 25. It is apparently unlikely that a woman will become a drinker in middle or old age if she has not already had drinking experience in her youth.

For women drinking more than minimally in the preceding year, Table 3 summarizes data on the prevalence and age of onset of relatively heavy drinking and adverse drinking consequences. Symptoms of alcohol dependence and drinking-related social or behavior problems were relatively common among women drinkers; a majority (57%) had experienced at least one problem consequence of drinking from a list of eleven. Problems and symptoms were typically first experienced and recognized early in adult life, although a few women could not recall when their first problem or symptom occurred (8% for the first problem, 11% for the first symptom). Chronic heavy drinking and general concerns about one's own drinking habits were less common and tended to develop later than specific experiences with problems or symptoms, and fewer women had any trouble recalling ages of onset. It is noteworthy that one out of five women drinkers had at some time worried about possibly having a drinking problem.

We compared different age cohorts of women to see how many of those women in each cohort who had begun drinking before age 25 had also engaged in heavier drinking, and how many had experienced adverse drinking consequences, before they were 25. The data in Table 3 suggest that early onsets of heavy drinking and of adverse consequences are more common among young women today than was true for older cohorts when they were young. This pattern may be interpreted several ways. It is possible that women forget some of their earlier experiences as they grow older. However, the contrasts between the two youngest cohorts seem too sharp to be explained only by forgetfulness, and even the oldest women did not forget how young they were when they started to drink. The data might in part reflect an actual acceleration of drinking experience and alcohol abuse among young women. Even though there has been little change in young women's drinking in the past ten years,[33,41] alcohol dependence symptoms have become more commonly reported by all women drinkers,[34] and some of the contrast between younger cohorts

Table 3. Percentages of Women Drinkers Reporting Various Drinking Experiences, Median Age of First Experience, and Percentages of Women by Age Group Reporting the First Experience Before Age 25[a]

Drinking Experience	Percent with Experience	Median Age of First Experience	First Experience Before Age 25, Among Those Drinking by Age 25: Percentage by Age Group of Respondents			
			25-34	35-49	50-64	65+
Drank Two or More Drinks Per Day, on the Average	22	29	8	5	2	0
Had a Social or Behavioral Problem as a Result of Drinking	57	23	48	17	9	0
Had a Symptom of Alcohol Dependence	40	22	36	10	7	0
Worried about Possibly Having a Drinking Problem	20	29	9	3	0	0
(Unweighted N)	(591)		(174)	(175)	(103)	(45)
(Weighted N)	(1125)		(315)	(356)	(202)	(84)

[a] Percentages and median ages are based on weighted data. N's here include respondents with missing data for particular items of information.

in Table 3 could stem from changes in behavior patterns before the 1970s. It also seems likely that the contrasts reflect cultural changes: young women may now drink more openly (exposing their drinking behavior to reactions from other people), other people may be less inclined now to protect or cover up young women's drinking behavior, and young women may be more conscious now of the potential effects of alcohol on their health and behavior.

One other piece of evidence that women do not simply forget their past drinking behavior is that they report *changes* in their drinking patterns over time. Even though the drinking history questions may not have detected gradual or temporary changes in drinking behavior, only 25% of current women drinkers said they had been drinking at the same level since they first began. Increases in drinking levels over time, with no reductions, were reported by 23% of the women drinkers; 10% reported reductions in drinking over time with no increases. The largest group of women drinkers, 42%, reported both increases and reductions in drinking during their lifetime drinking histories. This fluctuation in self-recognized levels indicates the importance of retrospective drinking histories, not only because the timing of increases and reductions in drinking may be related to other life experiences, but also because an adequate description of women's alcohol use in relation to other changes in their lives cannot be obtained from a single measure of *current* alcohol consumption, obtained once in a survey or only at the times of data collection in multiwave panel studies.

Relationships With Current vs. Maximum Lifetime Drinking Levels

To evaluate further the utility of the drinking history data, we compared how reported experiences of depression and reproductive problems were related to the detailed measure of current drinking levels versus how these experiences were related to the maximum level of consumption reported in the drinking histories. The comparison was limited to women who had been more than minimal drinkers in the preceding year, who had provided complete information about their drinking histories and current alcohol consumption, and who indicated that the most recent drinking level in their histories was also their current drinking behavior at the time of the survey. Because prior research had found that only very high levels of current consumption were related to adverse reproductive experiences,[39] and to allow exact comparisons, drinking levels were dichotomized to distinguish women who drank at least 6 drinks a day on 4 or more days a week (24 or more drinks per week) from other women drinkers who consumed less.

The associations (Yule's Q) between the two levels of current or maximum lifetime drinking and reproductive and depressive experiences are summarized Table 4. Yule's Q is the

Table 4. Relationships of High Levels of Current Drinking[a] and of Maximum Lifetime Drinking[b] with Lifetime Experience of Depression and Reproductive Problems

	Yule's Q	
Life Experience (Ever Had...)	Maximum Lifetime Drinking	Current Drinking
Two-Week or Longer Period of Depressed Mood	.545	.341
Depressive Episode[c]	.741	.329
Three or More Depressive Episodes	.822	.500
Suicide Attempt	.806	.472
Infertility for at Least One Year	.041	.151
	Among Women Ever Pregnant	
Miscarriage or Stillbirth	-.088	-.068
Premature Delivery	.230	.224
Baby with Birth Defect(s)	.023	.328

Note. Yule's Q is based on weighted data. For all women drinkers, unweighted N=506, weighted N=937. For women drinkers ever pregnant, unweighted N=380, weighted N=737. N's here include respondents with missing data for particular items of information.

[a] 24 drinks per week or more in the 30 days preceding the survey

[b] 6 or more drinks per day, 4 or more days per week

[c] Two-week or longer period of depressed mood plus 3 or more depressive symptoms

gamma statistic, a measure of association between ordinal variables, as applied to 2 × 2 contingency tables.[42]

At the threshold of 24 drinks per week, neither current heavy drinking nor the maximum lifetime drinking level was strongly related to experience with reproductive problems. The partial exception, a moderate relationship of current heavy drinking with a history of having a child with a birth defect, is based on a very small number of current heavy drinkers reporting the experience, and thus the value of Yule's Q is unstable.

Experiences with depression *were* related to current drinking but were related much more powerfully to maximum lifetime drinking levels. Of the women whose lifetime drinking had stayed below the 24 drinks/week threshold less than 3% reported ever attempting suicide, while of the women whose drinking had sometime exceeded the threshold, 25% at some time had also attempted suicide. Of the women whose lifetime drinking stayed below the threshold, only 10% had had three or more depressive episodes; of the women whose lifetime drinking at some point was above 24 drinks per week, 53% reported three or more depressive episodes in their lives. At least for the purpose of understanding the dynamics of depression in women, it seems very important to obtain as complete as possible a lifetime drinking history in addition to whatever information is obtained about current drinking behavior.

Time Sequences of Drinking and Health Problems

When women have histories of depression or reproductive problems and have also been heavy drinkers, it is essential to learn whether the heavy drinking began before or after the other experiences occurred. If heavy alcohol consumption among women is a major cause of depression and reproductive problems, then heavy-drinking women should already be drinking above some threshold level when these problems arise. If heavy drinking is more often a response to depression or reproductive problems (perhaps as self-medication for emotional distress), then the onset of heavy drinking should occur after the onset of the other problems. Time lags may also be important to consider, because long time lags could indicate weak or indirect relationships, or could signal that causal influences have to accumulate over time.

For women who reported experience with depression or reproductive problems and also experience with relatively heavy drinking, Table 5 summarizes relationships between ages of onset for drinking patterns and for the health problems. Onsets of two heavier-drinking levels are analyzed here: when a woman first began to consume an average of at least one drink a day, and when a woman began having six or more drinks in a day on at least four days a week. Findings for the second, more extreme level must be interpreted cautiously due to the small numbers of cases. Table 5 reports two time-ordered relationships: when a drinking level began *before* and *continued or increased through* the first experience with a health problem, and when a drinking level was reached *only after* the first experience with a health problem. The data base also included cases for which the time order was ambiguous, for example, because the onsets of both a health problem and above-threshold drinking occurred in the same year.

The majority of women in Table 5 reported that they began drinking relatively heavily only after experience with health problems. For most of these women, heavy drinking was *not* an antecedent of their first experience with depression or reproductive problems. The evidence against the hypothesis that heavy drinking precedes the onset of depression varied little among different age groups of respondents. In support of the reverse hypothesis that depression precedes heavier drinking, half of the women who reported both experiences began heavy drinking after the first depressive episode, at a median time lag of five years. Given the relatively large proportion of women (27%) reporting a ambiguous time-ordering of the two experiences, the data would also be consistent with an interpretation viewing both depressive episodes and heavy drinking as parts of a more general and prolonged process in which women are trying to cope or failing to cope with chronically distressful experiences.

Table 5 shows that when heavier drinking begins after the first reproductive problem, the drinking increase typically occurs a decade or more afterwards. One might argue that this time lag is an artifact of including cases in the "after" category no matter how long a drinking increase is delayed after

Table 5. Relationships Between Ages of Onset for Two Drinking Levels and for Depression and Reproductive Problems, Among Women Reporting Experiences with Both Drinking and Problems

Drinking Onset	Depressive Episode	Infertility	Miscarriage or Stillbirth	Premature Delivery	Baby with Birth Defect
One or More Drinks per Day Occurred...					
Before the First...	23%	22%	17%	22%	8%
After the First...	50%	51%	69%	61%	80%
Timing Ambiguous	27%	27%	14%	18%	11%
Median Years Before	5	4	4	*	*
Median Years After	5	10	9	13	12
(Unweighted N)	(137)	(39)	(74)	(29)	(15)
Six or More Drinks per Day, Four or More Days per Week Occurred...					
Before the First...	19%	31%	8%	11%	0%
After the First...	43%	69%	72%	62%	100%
Time Ambiguous	38%	0%	20%	27%	0%
Median Years Before	*	*	*	*	*
Median Years After	5	*	*	*	*
(Unweighted N)	(27)	(5)	(10)	(7)	(3)

Note. Percentages and median years are based on weighted data.

*N's too small to permit reliable estimates.

an earlier problem experience. The long time lag might be a warning that no causal relationship exists. However, the artifact interpretation cannot explain why women's drinking would change so much over their lifespans, or why women alcohol abusers report unusually high rates of past obstetrical and gynecological problems.[43] An alternative interpretation of the long time lags is that early reproductive problems may indirectly affect women's drinking later in life, by contributing to distress and dissatisfaction women feel about their lives (particularly relating to family life), distress and dissatisfaction which may be especially likely to lead to self-medicative drinking as women get closer to the end of their childbearing years.

CONCLUSIONS

Retrospective data regarding drinking in the general population are badly needed but are too often uncollected. The findings presented here from a national sample of women show some of the potential value of collecting and analyzing retrospective data on drinking and its possible antecedents and consequences. The findings make it clear that women's drinking levels are likely to change or fluctutate considerably during their lives. Experience with one or more drinking-related problems and symptoms of alcohol dependence was common among women drinkers and was likely to occur early in the lives of women who had become drinkers since the 1960s. Experience with depression was associated with higher levels of alcohol consumption in women's drinking histories, although heavy drinking was more likely to follow the onset of depression than to precede it. Heavy drinking was also more likely to follow than to predede initial experiences with reproductive problems, and typically developed a decade or so after these problems began. These findings do not mean that heavy drinking never causes or contributes to depression or reproductive disorders; there is ample evidence from animal and human studies, for example, that heavy drinking can lead to a variety of adverse reproductive consequences.[44-46] The findings presented here do suggest, however, that the reverse temporal sequence also occurs, perhaps even more often—that is, a sequence in which problems with depression or reproductive disorders precede and possibly contribute to the onset of heavy drinking.

These preliminary findings should make us aware of the needs for more complex time-ordered analyses. It is important to determine how much (if at all) certain levels of alcohol consumption increase the risks of various health problems over time, and vice versa. It is important to discover some of the more immediate precipitants of changes in women's drinking, and to learn to what extent the influences of life experiences on drinking depend on other characteristics of a woman's environment (such as her family, income, work, friends, etc.). And it is important to investigate how the dynamics of women's drinking and its consequences vary as women's ages vary. The point to be emphasized here is that retrospective data can make analyses such as these possible, if we invest a modest amount of effort in the questions we ask, and if we have a modest amount of faith in the memories of the people who answer our questions.

REFERENCES

1. Polich JM, Armor DJ, Braiker HB. The course of alcoholism. Four years after treatment. Santa Monica, Calif.: Rand Corporation, 1980.

2. Streissguth AP, Martin DC, Martin JC, Barr HM. The Seattle longitudinal prospective study on alcohol and pregnancy. Neurobehavioral Toxicology and Teratology 1981, 3:223–33.

3. Pettinati HM, Sugerman AA, DiDonato N, Maurer HS. The natural history of alcoholism over four years after treatment. Journal of Studies on Alcohol 1982; 43:201–15.

4. Aneshensel CS, Huba GJ. Depression, alcohol use, and smoking over one year: A four-wave longitudinal causal model. Journal of Abnormal Psychology 1983; 92:134–50.

5. Albert MS, Butters N, Brandt J. Memory for remote events in alcoholics. Journal of Studies on Alcohol 1980; 41:1071–81.

6. Field D. Retrospective reports by healthy intelligent elderly people of personal events of their adult lives. International Journal of Behavioral Development 1981; 4:77–97.

7. Brown GW, Harris T. Fall-off in the reporting of life events. Social Psychiatry 1982; 17:23–8.

8. Waldron I, Herold J, Dunn D. How valid are self-report measures for evaluating relationships between women's health and labor force participation? Women and Health 1982; 7:53–66.

9. Norbeck JS. Modification of life event questionnaires for use with female respondents. Research in Nursing and Health 1984; 7:61–71.

10. Cooper AM, Sobell MB, Sobell LC, Maisto SA. Validity of alcoholics' self-reports: Duration data. International Journal of the Addictions 1981; 16:401–6.

11. Polich JM. Epidemiology of alcohol abuse in military and civilian populations. American Journal of Public Health 1981; 71:1125–32.

12. Midanik L. The validity of self-reported alcohol consumption and alcohol problems: A literature review. British Journal of Addiction 1982; 77:357–82.

13. Bernadt MW. Drinking histories: Are they accurate? Neuropharmacology 1983; 22:571–2.

14. Skinner HA. Assessing alcohol use by patients in treatment. In: Smart RG et al., eds. Research advances in alcohol and drug problems (Vol.8). New York: Plenum Press, 1984:183–207.

15. Rohan WP. Quantitative dimensions of alcohol use for hospitalized problem drinkers. Diseases of the Nervous System 1976; 37:154–9.

16. Skinner HA, Sheu WJ. Reliability of alcohol use indices: The Lifetime Drinking History and the MAST. Journal of Studies on Alcohol 1982; 43:1157–70.

17. Little RE, Mandell W, Schultz FA. Consequences of retrospective measurement of alcohol consumption. Journal of Studies on Alcohol 1977; 38:1777–80.

18. Finney HC. Improving the reliability of retrospective survey measures: Results of a longitudinal field survey. Evaluation Review 1981; 5:207–29.

19. Paykel ES Methodological aspects of life events research. Journal of Psychosomatic Research 1983; 27:341–52.

20. Hannan MT, Tuma NB. Methods for temporal analysis. Annual Review of Sociology 1979; 5:303–28.

21. Aalen OO, Borgan O, Keiding N, Thormann J. Interaction between life history events: Nonparametric analysis for prospective and retrospective data in the presence of censoring. Scandinavian Journal of Statistics 1980; 7:161–71.

22 Teachman JD. Analyzing social processes: Life tables and proportional hazards models. Social Science Research 1983; 12:263–301.

23. Holubowycz OT. The roles of life events and support networks in the aetiology of female alcohol dependence. Australian Alcohol/Drug Review 1983; 2:40–4.

24. Reinecker H, Zauner H. Kritische Lebensereignisse als Risikofaktoren des Alkoholismus. Archiv fur Psychiatrie und Nervenkrankheiten 1983; 233:333–46.

25. Wells-Parker E, Miles S, Spencer B. Stress experiences and drinking histories of elderly drunken-driving offenders. Journal of Studies on Alcohol 1983; 44:429–37.

26. Morrissey ER, Schuckit MA. Stressful life events and alcohol problems among women seen at a detoxication center. Journal of Studies on Alcohol 1978; 39:1559–76.

27. Tarter RE. Psycho-social history, minimal brain dysfunction, and differential drinking patterns of male alcoholics. Journal of Clinical Psychology 1982; 38:867–73.

28. Stockwell T, Small P, Hodgson R, Canter S. Alcohol dependence and phobic anxiety states II A retrospective study. British Journal of Psychiatry 1984; 144:58–63.

29. Cahalan D. Problem drinkers: A national survey. San Francisco: Jossey-Bass, 1970.

30. Clark WB, Midanik L. Alcohol use and alcohol problems among U.S. adults: Results of the 1979 national survey. In: Alcohol consumption and related problems (Alcohol and Health Monograph No. 1, U.S. Department of Health and Human Services Publication No. ADM-82-1190). Washington D.C.: U.S. Government Printing Office, 1982:3–52.

31 U.S. Department of Commerce, Bureau of the Census. Statistical abstract of the United States (101st edition). Washington, D.C.: U.S. Government Printing Office, 1980.

32. Davis JA. General Social Surveys, 1972–1980: Cumulative codebook. Chicago: National Opinion Research Center, 1980.

33. Wilsnack RW, Wilsnack SC, Klassen AD. Women's drinking and drinking

problems: Patterns from a 1981 national survey. American Journal of Public Health 1984; 74:1231–8.

34. Wilsnack SC, Wilsnack RW, Klassen AD. Epidemiological research on women's drinking, 1978–1984. In: Proceedings of the National Research Conference on Women and Alcohol (University of Washington, Seattle, May 1984). Washington, D.C.: U.S. Government Printing Office, in press.

35. Robins LN. Washington University Followup Interview (interview questionnaires for community survey of alcohol use and psychiatric disorder). St. Louis: Washington University School of Medicine, October 1980, February 1981

36. Miller Communications, Inc. Health history questionnaire: Gynecology screen. Norwalk, Ct.: Miller Communications, 1976.

37. OB-GYN, Inc. Health questionnaire. Bloomington, Ind.: OB-GYN, Inc., 1980.

38. National Institute of Mental Health. The NIMH Diagnostic Interview Schedule (DIS). Version I: 2-14-79. Version III: 2-5-81. Rockville, Md.: NIMH.

39. Wilsnack SC, Klassen AD, Wilsnack RW. Drinking and reproductive dysfunction among women in a 1981 national survey. Alcoholism: Clinical and Experimental Research 1984; 8:451–8.

40. Williams G, Aitken S, Malin H. Validity/reliability study of self-reported drinking. Working Paper of the Alcohol Epidemiologic Data System, Washington, D.C., April 1983.

41. Thompson KM, Wilsnack RW. Drinking and drinking problems among female adolescents: Patterns and influences. In: Wilsnack SC, Beckman LJ, eds. Alcohol problems in women: Antecedents, consequences, and intervention. New York: Guilford Press, 1984:37–65.

42. Blalock HM. Social statistics (Revised second edition). New York McGraw-Hill, 1979.

43. Wilsnack SC. Alcohol, sexuality, and reproductive dysfunction in women. In: Abel EL, ed. Fetal alcohol syndrome (Vol. 2: Human studies). Boca Raton, Fla.: CRC Press, 1982:21–46.

44. Streissguth AP, Landesman-Dwyer S, Martin JC, Smith DW. Teratogenic effects of alcohol in humans and animals. Science 1980; 209:353–61

45. Abel EL, ed. Fetal alcohol syndrome, Vols. 1–3. Boca Raton, Fla · CRC Press. 1982.

46. Little RE, Ervin CH. Alcohol use and reproduction. In: Wilsnack SC, Beckman LJ, eds. Alcohol problems in women: Antecedents, consequences, and intervention. New York: Guilford Press, 1984: 155–88.

Substance Use Among Females in New York State: Catching Up With the Males

Elisabeth Kaestner, PhD
Blanche Frank, PhD
Rozanne Marel, PhD
James Schmeidler, PhD

ABSTRACT. Epidemiologic surveys of the New York State population over the past several years show substance use rates for females that are approaching the higher use rates for males. Surveys of the secondary school population show similar rates of use for girls and boys over time as well as a similar intensity of involvement. Surveys of adults show a dramatic increase of use for females, ages 18 to 34 years, in recent years, and a more modest increase for females, ages 35 years and older. An analysis of substance use by sex, age, marital status and employment identifies disparate rates of use among subgroups. For instance, among younger adults, single full-time employed women have considerably higher rates of use than housewives for illicit substances as well as psychoactive prescription drugs used medically as well as nonmedically.

INTRODUCTION

The role of women in our society has been changing radically in the past twenty years, and these changes have become increasingly more accepted and established. For example, it is not unusual at this time for women to return to work after bearing children and for employers to arrange for part-time positions. Similarly, the double standard of prescribed mores and behaviors for men and women has relaxed, though not

Dr. Kaestner, formerly associated with the New York State Division of Substance Services, is now a psychologist in private practice in New York City. Drs. Frank, Marel, and Schmeidler are research scientists with the New York State Division of Substance Abuse Services, 55 West 125 St., New York, NY 10027.

29

disappeared. Women also have gained entry into previously all-male professions such as the military and the police, and they have become visible in traditionally all-male sports e.g., the marathon. Legal battles have been fought and are being won regarding equal rights in such areas as membership in private clubs or societies. Women also have become more accepted in the financial world as credit risks and in top management positions. In short, women have been moving into positions that have been traditionally more male.

There is some documentation that the once sharply distinguished patterns of male and female drug use are also blurring. Prather and Fidell (1978),[1] in a review of the literature, concluded that sex differences were rapidly disappearing and that the differences were especially small among the younger users. A recent extensive review article on sex differences in psychoactive drug use by Ferrence and Whitehead (1980)[2] challenges this position by concluding that males invariably had higher use rates than females for illicit drugs and the nonmedical use of prescription drugs, a pattern which has been stable over the past years. However, these authors also caution the reader about limitations in their data sources.

The present paper presents prevalence data for male and female substance use from several cross-sectional surveys of one large geographical area. Rather than inquiring about the use of several single drugs, attempts were made to assess the use of all relevant illegal and legal psychoactive drugs, used medically and nonmedically. Since surveys were repeated at several year intervals, and were conducted by the same research team, using similar methods of assessment and analysis, the findings lend themselves to trend analyses in substance use among females and males.

METHODOLOGY

The New York State Division of Substance Abuse Services is responsible for assessing the extent of substance use in the New York State population. As a result, a variety of statewide surveys of the population are periodically conducted. These include surveys of secondary school students and surveys of the household population. These specific surveys will provide the major findings presented in this paper.

Comparable secondary school surveys were conducted

throughout New York State in 1978[3] with 35,300 participants and in 1983[4] with 27,400 participants in grades seven through 12. The vast majority of students ranged in age from 12 years through 17 years. The self-administered questionnaires that the students completed were very similar for both years with questions that probed the use of a variety of illicit substances and psychoactive prescription drugs used nonmedically. The survey findings for the separate, stratified random samples were statistically projected to reflect findings for the state's 1.8 million secondary school students in 1978 and the state's 1.5 million secondary school students in 1983.

Household surveys were conducted throughout the state in 1975–1976[5] with face-to-face interviews of 11,410 household residents and in 1981[6] with telephone interviews of 3,487 household residents. Pretesting for the latter survey compared telephone interviews with face-to-face interviews, and similar rates of response and drug usage were found for these two methods. Although the 1975–1976 study surveyed the household population aged 14 years and older and the 1981 study surveyed the household population aged 12 years and older, the household findings presented here will highlight findings for the adult sub-population aged 18 years and older. The content of the interviews for the two household surveys were similar, except that the 1981 questionnaire probed the medical use of psychoactive prescription drugs in addition to the nonmedical use of these drugs (i.e., use beyond the prescribed dose and/or obtained from a nonmedical source) and the use of illicit substances; the 1975–1976 survey inquired only into the nonmedical use of psychoactive prescription drugs and the use of illicit substances. The household survey findings for the 1975–1976 stratified, random sample of 9,500 respondents, 18 years and older, were statistically projected to reflect findings for the state's then 12.1 million residents in that age range. Similarly, findings for the 1981 stratified random sample of 2,972 comparable respondents were statistically projected to reflect findings for the state's 12.5 million residents, 18 years and older in that year.

The section that follows introduces the findings by presenting a broad overview of substance use by sex for several age groups for 1979 and 1984. The basic data sources for these estimates and projections are the secondary school surveys and household surveys discussed above as well as a college

survey conducted in 1979.[7] Estimates of substance use were
made based on these survey findings for the mutually exclu-
sive subsets of the population, and projections were made for
1979 and 1984 based on the rates of change found for the two
school surveys and the two household surveys.

In addition, this overview includes special estimates made
for narcotic use. Since surveys of school populations and
household populations do not provide an effective basis for
sampling narcotic users, another strategy for estimating the
prevalence of illicit narcotic use was devised. This methodology was based on regression analysis that related New York
City Narcotics Register estimates with indirect indicators of
narcotic use.[8]

RESULTS

Overview of Trends in Nonmedical Substance Use
Among Women and Men: 1979-1984

The summary overview of substance use presented in Table
1 for the five year period between 1979 and 1984 shows some
interesting trends and some interesting contrasts by age between females and males in New York State. Overall, both
sexes have had increasing experience with the use of illicit
substances and the nonmedical use of psychoactive prescription drugs. Although a higher proportion of males have used
these substances in their lifetime, females show a greater increase in rates of "ever" use in the past five years—an increase of eight percentage points for females (from 29 percent
to 37 percent), as well as an increase of six percentage points
for males (from 40 percent to 46 percent).

By age group, the most important change is found among
younger adult women, ages 18 to 34 years. In 1979, it was
estimated that 49 percent of these women had at one time
been users. By 1984, the rate of lifetime use was estimated to
increase to 63 percent, an increase of 14 percentage points.
For men, the changes were relatively small, from 63 percent
in 1979 to 69 percent in 1984. Of interest is the fact that the
increase for women was mainly in "prior" use or use in the
past but not continued into the immediate past six months.
Women's prior use had increased 10 percentage points com-

TABLE 1. RECENCY OF NONMEDICAL SUBSTANCE USE[a] AMONG NEW YORK STATE RESIDENTS, BY SEX AND AGE, 1979 and 1984

	1979		1984	
	Females	Males	Females	Males
Total Population: Ages 12 Years and Older	(N=7,672,800)	(N=6,783,300)	(N=7,673,900)	(N=6,910,400)
Never Used	71%	60%	63%	54%
Ever Used	29	40	37	46
Prior Use[b]	13%	16%	19%	21%
Recent Use[c]	16	24	18	25
Youth: Ages 12-17	(N=917,900)	(N=938,100)	(N=780,100)	(N=809,300)
Never Used	39%	35%	37%	36%
Ever Used	61	65	63	64
Prior Use[b]	10%	10%	16%	16%
Recent Use[c]	51	55	47	48
Younger Adults: Ages 18-34	(N=2,534,000)	(N=2,374,800)	(N=2,564,600)	(N=2,497,600)
Never Used	51%	37%	31%	37%
Ever Used	49	63	63	69
Prior Use[b]	24%	25%	34%	30%
Recent Use[c]	25	38	29	39
Older Adults: Ages 35 and Older	(N=4,220,900)	(N=3,470,400)	(N=4,329,200)	(N=3,603,500)
Never Used	89%	83%	83%	75%
Ever Used	11	17	17	25
Prior Use[b]	8%	11%	12%	15%
Recent Use[c]	3	6	5	10

[a]Refers to the use of any one or more illicit substances and/or the nonmedical use of psychoactive prescription drugs.

[b]Use in the past, but not in the previous six months.

[c]Use in the past six months.

pared to five percentage points for men. In fact, prior use among women in 1984 (34 percent) exceeded prior use among men (30 percent). When recent substance use (i.e., use in the past six months) is considered, the gap in use rates between young adult women and men is narrowing. In 1979 there was a difference of 13 percentage points (25 percent for females and 38 percent for males) compared to 10 percentage points in 1984 (29 percent for females and 39 percent for males), although recent use rates among men continue to be substantially higher than among women.

Older adults, ages 35 years and older, show increased substance use as well, but the changes are less dramatic than those found among younger adults. Although the vast majority of older adults have never had experience with nonmedical substance use, lifetime rates among older men increased eight percentage points (from 17 percent to 25 percent) in the past five years and use among older women increased six percentage points (from 11 percent to 17 percent). Similarly, the trend in prior use and recent use rates shows a general pattern of increasing use. Although rates for males exceed those for females, rates for both sexes have increased at a similar pace.

The importance of analyzing substance use rates for the sexes by age is borne out by the findings for youths, ages 12 years through 17 years, that show still another pattern of substance use over time. Here, the five year trend looks stable with little difference in use rates for girls and boys. In 1979, lifetime use rates were 61 percent for females and 65 percent for males; in 1984, the rates were 63 percent and 64 percent, respectively. Interestingly, recent use rates may have declined for both sexes among youth while comparable use rates have increased for other age groups.

Despite the diverse patterns among the several age groups the overall trend appears to be a general increase in past and present nonmedical substance use, a slight increase in recent use, and a converging of rates for the sexes. For youths, the trend has been most stable over the past five years with substance use rates that are most similar for females and males. For younger adults, the trend has shown particular increases for women leading to a converging of rates for lifetime use for the sexes. For older adults, the trend is increasing for both men and women, but the rates are not converging and substance use rates for men continue to exceed those for women.

The sections that follow look more closely at females and males in the individual age group and the subpopulations within them. The next section begins with girls and boys in the secondary school population, their rates of use of specific substances and other substance using behaviors.

Nonmedical Substance Use Among Female and Male
Secondary School Students: 1978 and 1983

As already indicated, females and males among youths have the highest recent substance use rates in the population. Table 2 shows these rates for the more popular substances used by

TABLE 2. RECENT NONMEDICAL USE OF SELECTED SUBSTANCES AMONG NEW YORK STATE
STUDENTS IN GRADES 7 THROUGH 12, BY SEX, 1978 and 1983[a]

Selected Substances	1978		1983	
	Females	Males	Females	Males
	(N=901,900)	(N=906,500)	(N=772,800)	(N=762,200)
Marijuana	43%	47%	33%	36%
Cocaine	6	8	8	12
PCP (Angel Dust)	8	10	2	4
Other Hallucinogens[b]	4	7	5	7
Stimulants[c]	11	10	18	16
Tranquilizers[c]	9	7	7	7
Sedatives[c]	7	7	8	9

[a]Recent Use refers to use since school began in September 1977 for the 1978 findings and use since school began in September 1982 for the 1983 findings.

[b]Other Hallucingens include substances such as LSD, mescaline and psilocybin.

[c]Refers only to nonmedical use, defined as use "on your own, without a doctor telling you to." Stimulants include amphetamines and prescription diet pills; tranquilizers include Valium and Librium, sedatives include barbiturates, methaqualone and Tuinal.

Note: The (N's) on which percentages are based may vary.

the secondary school population in the approximate six months prior to the 1978 survey and prior to the 1983 survey.

In general, females and males follow the same trends. For instance, in the five year period, rates of recent marijuana use and PCP use have declined for both sexes while rates of recent cocaine use and nonmedical use of stimulants have increased for both. Rates of recent use of hallucinogens, such as LSD, mescaline and psilocybin, have been relatively stable as have the nonmedical use of tranquilizers and sedatives.

Use rates for specific substances are generally similar for females and males, although small differences in patterns do persist. First, use rates for illicit substances, such as marijuana, cocaine and PCP, are consistently higher for males. In fact, use rates for cocaine may be widening. In 1978, the difference in cocaine rates for females and males was two percent, in 1983 the difference was four percent. A second pattern shows that nonmedical use rates for psychoactive prescription drugs, such as stimulants and tranquilizers, are either slightly higher for females or about the same for both sexes. The nonmedical use of stimulants appears to be increasingly more popular, with females showing greater involvement. While questions were explicitly asked for prescription stimulants, it is possible that use of over-the-counter diet pills contributed somewhat to the increasing rates.

A look at drug behavior that indicates seriousness of involvement reveals similar rates, or, if anything, a narrowing of differences between the sexes. For example, polydrug use shows a converging of rates. In 1978, 30 percent of the females and 34 percent of the males reported this practice in the previous six months; in 1983, the comparable rates were 27 percent and 29 percent, respectively. Similarly, when the number of substances recently used and the frequency of use are compared over time, a narrowing of differences is also seen. In 1978, nine percent of females and 12 percent of males were considered at least substantial users.* The comparable rates for 1983 were nine percent of females and 11 percent of males.

Of interest is the fact that the 1983 survey found small differences in rates of substance using behavior between females and males but found large differences between the sexes for other problem-causing behavior. For instance, in addition to similar rates of substance use, 12 percent of females report being high on marijuana during school in the month prior to the survey compared to 15 percent of the males. Nevertheless, girls receive D's or fail at a lower rate (three percent for females vs. seven percent of males), girls are less likely to be sent to a school administrator because of conduct (21 percent vs. 37 percent, respectively, in the previous six months), and girls are less likely to have someone contacted from home because of their behavior (11 percent vs. 18 percent, respectively, in the previous six months). Although a variety of substance abuse behaviors occur at similar rates for girls and boys, other problem behaviors seem to occur at lower rates for girls than for boys.

Nonmedical Substance Use Among Adult Female and Male Household Residents: 1975-1976 and 1981

This part of the analysis looks more closely at adult females and males. Findings for nonmedical substance use among

---

*Defined as use of at least seven illicit substances and/or psychoactive prescription drugs used nonmedically in the past six months; or the use of marijuana at least 40 times in the past month; or the use of a substance other than marijuana at least four times in the past month.

adults in the 1975-1976 and in the 1981 household surveys show general increases for both sexes over time and particular increases for those 18 to 34 years of age, and especially the females among them. The following discussion first focuses on the younger adults and then turns to the older adults.

Younger Adults: 18 to 34 years

Table 3 presents recent use rates for the more popular illicit substances and psychoactive prescription drugs used nonmedically in the 1975-1976 and 1981 surveys. In general, the rates of use increased markedly for younger adults. Recent prevalence of marijuana use among the younger women increased from 16 percent to 20 percent. For younger men, the rate remained stable (31 percent and 30 percent). Although rates of nonmedical tranquilizer use remained remarkably constant, recent use of cocaine and stimulants increased dramatically and at a similar rate for both sexes.

Other indications show the pattern of increasing involvement with substance use for younger adults, with younger women showing particular increases. For instance, polydrug use has increased among younger women. In 1975-1976, 13 percent of younger women used marijuana with alcohol in the previous six months; in 1981 the comparable rate was 16 percent. For younger men, the practice decreased from 29 percent to 25 percent during the same time period. Use of other combinations has increased to a similar extent among younger women and men. While one percent of women used marijuana and cocaine in 1975-1976, four percent did so in 1981. For comparably aged men, use of marijuana and cocaine increased from two percent to eight percent.

Furthermore, incidence data support the pattern of increasing involvement among younger adults, with particular increases among younger women. In the 1975-1976 survey, there was a higher proportion of men than women who reported the first use of marijuana in the previous year (two percent of the men compared to one percent of the women). The 1981 survey found a higher proportion of women than men starting marijuana use in the previous year (two percent of the women compared to one percent of the men). Use of other drugs, such as cocaine, spread equally among younger

TABLE 3. RECENT USE OF SELECTED SUBSTANCES AMONG NEW YORK STATE
HOUSEHOLD RESIDENTS, BY AGE AND SEX, 1975-1976 and 1981[a]

| | Ages 18 to 34 | | | | Ages 35 and Older | | | |
| | 1975-1976 | | 1981 | | 1975-1976 | | 1981 | |
Selected Substances	Females (N=2,129,000)	Males (N=1,965,000)	Females (N=2,409,000)	Males (N=2,297,000)	Females (N=4,315,000)	Males (N=3,657,000)	Females (N=4,226,000)	Males (N=3,523,000)
Marijuana	10%	31%	20%	30%	1%	3%	2%	4%
Cocaine	2	4	6	10	*	1	*	2
Stimulants[b]	2	3	5	3	*	*	1	1
Tranquilizers[b]	2	2	2	2	1	1	1	1

[a]Recent use refers to use in the six months prior to the survey.

[b]Refers only to nonmedical use, defined as use other than according to a physician's direction, i.e., in amounts beyond the prescribed dose and/or obtained from a nonmedical source. Stimulants include amphetamines and diet pills; Tranquilizers include Valium and Librium.

*Less than 0.5%.

Note: The (N's) on which percentages are based may vary.

women and men. Three percent, each, started using cocaine in the previous year.

When intensity of substance use is considered, the increase for the younger adult females becomes particularly apparent. The prevalence of regular substance use* for younger women increased from six percent in 1975-1976 to 11 percent in 1981 whereas regular use for younger men remained at a stable rate of 17 and 18 percent.

The 1981 household survey also asked respondents whether their substance use ever caused problems in the areas of family, friends, work or school, health, accidents, or the law. Overall, 14 percent of younger women and 17 percent of younger men report having had problems in any of these areas. When specific areas are considered, nine percent of women report problems with work or school compared to 10 percent of men; six percent of women and men both report health problems; seven percent of women report problems in relationships with family or friends compared to 10 percent of the men. Younger men more often than younger women say they have experienced trouble with the law as a result of using drugs nonmedically; five percent of the men vs. one percent of the women.

The 1981 survey also asked users whether they saw themselves as dependent on any of the drugs they were using. Men more often report dependency on illegal drugs, whereas dependency on prescription drugs used nonmedically is similar for women and men. Among younger adults, four percent of men and one percent of women report dependency on marijuana, and two percent of men and one percent of women on other illicit drugs. Dependency on prescription drugs is one percent, each, for men and women.

Older Adults: 35 Years and Older

Although rates of substance use are considerably lower for older adults than for younger adults, trends are similar for both age groups. While older women and men are less likely to use drugs nonmedically than younger adults, the slight in-

---

*Defined for adults as the recent nonmedical use of at least three different substances or at least the use of marijuana several times per week in the past month.

creases of use during the past years have been observed among both sexes, as can be seen for marijuana use and stimulant use (Table 3).

Other indications of involvement with substance use are small compared to younger adults. For instance, polydrug use or combinational use is not at all common. In 1975-1976, one percent of older women and three percent of older men had reported the use of marijuana and alcohol in the past six months; in 1981 the rates were similar—one percent and four percent, respectively. The percentage of older women and older men who were at least regular substance users in 1975-1976 were one and two percent, respectively; the comparable percentages in 1981 were less than one-half of one percent and one percent.

With respect to problems in everyday life related to substance use, in 1981 only one percent of the older women and two percent of older men indicated such difficulties. Among older adults, dependency on illicit drugs or prescription drugs was about one percent for men and less than one-half of one percent for women.

Patterns of Medical and Nonmedical Substance Use
Among Selected Subgroups of Adult Females and Males: 1981

With current roles for adult women ranging broadly, this section takes the analysis beyond the variables of just sex and age, and examines in addition variables that imply life style, which in turn may have consequences for substance use. Marital status and the combined effect of marital status and selected aspects of employment permit a view of the married or the single (i.e., never married, widowed, separated and divorced) as well as married housewives and the single full-time employed, both males and females.

Furthermore, this section looks at two patterns of substance use. Table 4 presents findings for the medical and nonmedical use of psychoative prescription drugs in the previous year,* and Table 5 presents rates for selected illicit drugs and

---

*Due to cyclical medical use of psychoactive prescription drugs. a year was used as a time reference in the analysis of these findings. The psychoactive prescription drugs include tranquilizers, such as Valium and Librium; sedatives, such as barbiturates and methaqualone: stimulants, such as amphetamines and diet pills; anti-depressants, such as Elavil and Imipramine; analgesics, such as Demerol and Darvon.

psychoative prescription drugs used nonmedically in the previous six months. These findings are presented only for 1981 when questions dealing with both medical and nonmedical use were asked.

Younger Adults: 18 to 34 years

When psychoactive prescription drug use is considered among younger adults, overall rates for single females and single males are higher than those for married females and married males (Table 4). Similarly, comparable rates for single full-time employed females and males are higher than the rates for housewives. In fact, the discrepancy in rates of psychoactive prescription drug use for the housewife (27 percent) and the single full-time employed female (45 percent) is the largest when comparing younger adult females, and, perhaps unexpectedly, with the housewife having the lower rate.

The medical use of psychoactive prescription drugs is highest for females irrespective of marital status and selected employment status with the single female (27 percent) and the single full-time employed female (29 percent) showing the highest rates of use. When, however, nonmedical use is considered, single males (13 percent) and single full-time employed males (11 percent) have the highest rates. Single females and single full-time employed females also show the highest rates of both medical and nonmedical use.

The particular categories of psychoactive prescription drugs used by these subpopulations were very similar. Analgesics were the most popular, irrespective of sex, marital status and selected aspects of employment, followed by stimulants and then tranquilizers.

When nonmedical use of selected substances in the recent past is considered (Table 5), the "singles" have by far the highest rates of use with males exceeding females. Overall, 33 percent of single females have used a substance nonmedically in the previous six months compared to 11 percent of the married females, 19 percent of the married males and nine percent of the housewives. The single males with an overall 42 percent use rate have the highest prevalence of all.

Little difference exists between the rates of use of selected substances whether marital status is considered alone or in

TABLE 4. ONE-YEAR MEDICAL AND NONMEDICAL USE[a] OF PSYCHOACTIVE PRESCRIPTION DRUGS[b]
AMONG NEW YORK STATE HOUSEHOLD RESIDENTS, BY AGE AND SEX, 1981

A. BY MARITAL STATUS

| | Ages 18 to 34 | | | | Ages 35 and Older | | | |
| | Married | | Single[c] | | Married | | Single[c] | |
	Females (N=1,137,000)	Males (N=1,008,000)	Females (N=1,190,000)	Males (N=1,191,000)	Females (N=2,495,000)	Males (N=2,610,000)	Females (N=1,711,000)	Males (N=887,000)
Any Use in Past Year	29%	24%	44%	39%	32%	22%	28%	27%
Medical Use Only	23	16	27	20	30	18	26	23
Nonmedical Use Only	3	5	6	13	1	4	2	4
Both Medical and Nonmedical Use	3	3	11	6	1	*	*	*

Table 4, cont.

B. BY MARITAL STATUS AND EMPLOYMENT

	Ages 18 to 34			Ages 35 and Older		
	Married Housewife[d]	Single[c] Full-time Employed		Married Housewife[d]	Single[c] Full-time Employed	
	Females (N=479,000)	Females (N=658,000)	Males (N=703,000)	Females (N=947,000)	Females (N=499,000)	Males (N=404,000)
Any Use in Past Year	27%	45%	36%	33%	23%	37%
Medical Use Only	20	29	18	33	21	30
Nonmedical Use Only	4	6	11	*	2	7
Both Medical and Nonmedical Use	3	10	7	*	*	*

[a]Medical Use refers to use according to a physician's directions in the year prior to the survey; Nonmedical Use refers to use beyond the prescribed dose and/or obtained from a nonmedical source in the year prior to the survey.

[b]Psychoactive Prescription Drugs include tranquilizers, such as Valium and Librium; sedatives such as barbiturates and methaqualone; stimulants such as amphetamines and diet pills; anti-depressants such as Elavil and Imipramine; analgesics such as Demerol and Darvon.

[c]Single is defined as never married, divorced, separated or widowed.

[d]Housewife is defined as a married female who is currently "keeping house." There were too few male counterparts in the sample to present comparable findings.

*Less than 0.5%.

Note: The (N's) on which percentages are based may vary.

TABLE 5. RECENT NONMEDICAL USE OF SELECTED SUBSTANCES AMONG NEW YORK STATE HOUSEHOLD RESIDENTS, BY AGE AND SEX, 1981[a]

A. BY MARITAL STATUS

| | Ages 18 to 34 | | | | Ages 35 and Older | | | |
| | Married | | Single[b] | | Married | | Single[b] | |
Selected Substances	Females (N=1,137,000)	Males (N=1,008,000)	Females (N=1,190,000)	Males (N=1,191,000)	Females (N=2,495,000)	Males (N=2,610,000)	Females (N=1,711,000)	Males (N=687,000)
Any Recent Use[c]	11%	19%	33%	42%	3%	5%	4%	12%
Marijuana	8	18	30	38	1	3	2	7
Cocaine	1	2	3	15	*	*	*	4
Stimulants[d]	3	2	6	12	1	2	*	1
Tranquilizers[d]	2	1	2	2	1	*	*	1

Table 5, cont.

B. BY MARITAL STATUS AND EMPLOYMENT

	Ages 18 to 34			Ages 35 and Older		
	Housewife[e]	Single Full-time Employed		Housewife[e]	Single Full-time Employed	
Selected Substances	Females (N=479,000)	Females (N=658,000)	Males (N=703,000)	Females (N=947,000)	Females (N=499,000)	Males (N=404,000)
Any Recent Use[c]	9%	32%	41%	*	4%	24%
Marijuana	6	28	39	*	2	12
Cocaine	1	12	18	*	1	8
Stimulants[d]	4	8	10	*	1	1
Tranquilizers[d]	1	4	2	*	*	1

a Recent Use refers to use in the six months prior to the survey.

b Single is defined as never married, divorced, separated or widowed.

c Any Recent Use includes the use of any one or more illicit substances and/or the nonmedical use of psychoactive prescription drugs.

d Refers only to nonmedical use, defined as use other than according to a physician's direction, i.e., in amounts beyond the prescribed dose and/or obtained from a nonmedical source. Stimulants include amphetamines and diet pills; tranquilizers include Valium and Librium.

e Housewife is defined as a married female who is currently "keeping house." There were too few male counterparts in the sample to present comparable findings.

* Less than 0.5%.

Note: The (N's) on which percentages are based may vary.

45

combination with selected employment characteristics. An exception is in rates of cocaine use. Single, full-time employed females and males have higher rates of cocaine use than all single females and males. For instance, 12 percent of single full-time employed females used cocaine in the six months prior to the survey compared to nine percent of all single females.

Older Adults: 35 Years and Older

Among the older adults, psychoactive prescription drugs are used somewhat differently than among the younger adults. When considering marital status alone, married females show the highest overall rate of use (32 percent). When employment factors are considered, single full-time employed males show the highest total rate (37 percent). Although housewives show the highest rate of medical use (33 percent), the relatively high nonmedical use among single full-time employed males (seven percent) in addition to medical use (30 percent) give them the highest rate of use of psychoactive prescription drugs. Interestingly, the single full-time employed female among the older adults has the lowest overall rate of use.

Like younger adults the particular category of psychoactive prescription drugs favored by older adults is analgesics. Unlike the stimulants favored by younger adults, the second preferred category is tranquilizers.

When nonmedical use of illicit and/or prescription drugs is considered, single full-time employed males (24 percent) have by far the highest rates of use among older adults, followed by single males (12 percent) and married males (five percent). Overall rates of use for single females (four percent) and married females (three percent) are very similar. In general however, illicit substance use is considerably lower among older adults than among younger adults.

DISCUSSION

The basis for most of the findings presented in this paper are direct surveys of the population. Although such epidemiological surveys depend on self-reported information and do miss important subgroups in the population (e.g., the home-less and school dropouts, which overrepresent males), they are the best available strategy for assessing the prevalence of substance use in the general population.

Consistent with Prather and Fidell (1978),[1] the present find-ings show a narrowing of the discrepancy in substance use rates between the sexes with use rates for females increasing and approaching the higher rates for males. The trends for individual age groups, however, differ. For youths, rates for females and males approximate each other and have been stable for the five years between surveys. For younger adults, rates for females have made the most dramatic increase, espe-cially for prior use. For older adults, the rates for females have increased somewhat but the discrepancy in rates be-tween females and males remains almost unchanged, a finding more consistent with the conclusions of Ferrence and White-head (1980).[2] The powerful role of age in accounting for dif-ferences in drug use rates among males and females was also noted by Pihl, Marinier, Lapp and Drake (1982)[9] and Ver-brugge (1982).[10]

The analysis also shows the importance of going beyond the relationship between substance use and age and examining the relationship between substance use, age and statuses, such as marital status and employment. The contrast in use rates for housewives and single full-time employed females shows most dramatically how widely rates for females may vary. When psychoactive prescription drugs are considered, not only are the rates of *any use* for single full-time employed younger adult females higher than rates for comparably aged housewives, but the rates for single full-time employed older adult females are lower than rates for comparably aged house-wives. When the use of illicit substances is considered, the rates of use for these single full-time employed females are at least four times the rates for the younger adult housewives. Furthermore, substance use rates for single younger adult females far exceed rates for married younger adult males and come closer to those for single younger adult males, whose rates of use are the highest of the subgroups analyzed.

The findings presented here also point to possible miscon-ceptions that may be held about substance use among females as well as males. First, prescription drug misuse has been commonly attributed to females, particularly housewives.[11] Consistent with this notion are the findings that older women, especially housewives, use prescription drugs. However, they use them only as prescribed by a doctor and from legal sourcs, i.e., medically. Nonmedical use, or use of illegal drugs is negligible. Among younger adult women, however, medical use is far less common, even among housewives, and nonmedical use is more prevalent. In comparisons between sexes, however, the findings still show that males' prescription drug use is almost equal to that of females. Among younger adults, in fact, single males have the highest nonmedical use rates; among older adults single full-time employed males have the highest rates.

Second, it is often assumed that males, particularly younger adult males have the highest use rates of illicit substances. Although this is indeed the case, differentiation needs to be made between single and married males among the younger adults. Rates of illicit substance use for the single males far exceed rates for married males, and, as stated above, even the single younger adult females have rates that far exceed the comparably aged married males.

A final misconception may have to do with a perception that females are not likely to be substance abuscrs, a notion which may impede efforts to identify this and other problems among females. It is interesting to find that although girls and boys show substance use rates and intensity of involvement that are very similar, girls report a considerably lower prevalence of encounters with school and law enforcement personnel over their substance using behavior. Of course, girls may be extremely discrete in their behavior, or, perhaps, the expectation that females are not involved in problem behaviors such as substance use may result in problems that go undetected, biases that persist, and consequences that result from a delayed response to the problem.

Finally, the present findings are suggestive of how change is taking place. One might hypothesize that by the 1980s in New York State, the catching up with males has already occurred for the youthful females, that it is most actively taking place among younger adult females, and has only modestly taken place among older adult females. In the past years, of course, the youthful females of the late 1970s have become younger adults in the 1980s as have younger adult females become older adults, bringing with them life experience from an earlier period of time (e.g., Prior Use), and, perhaps, an acceptance of substance use that now ripples through the several age groups discussed here.

CONCLUSIONS

Survey findings for New York State and the analyses presented here indicate a need for research that identifies the subgroups among the sexes that are most at risk of substance use. In addition, an understanding of the etiology of substance use and other correlates of use for these subgroups might help find specific ways in which the problem may be addressed. In any case, it is clear that in New York State the problem of substance use among youth and younger adults has become almost as widespread among females as it is among males.

REFERENCES

1. Prather, J.E. and Fidell, L.S. Drug Use and Abuse Among Women: An Overview. Int. J Addict, 13(6), 863–885, 1978.
2. Ferrence, R.G. and Whitehead, P.C. Sex Differences in Psychoactive Drug Use. Recent Epidemiology In: Kalant, O.J. (Ed). Alcohol and Drug Problems in Women. Research Advances in Alcohol and Drug Problems. Vol. 5, 125–201. New York: Plenum Press, 1980.
3. New York State Division of Substance Abuse Services. Substance Use Among New York State Public and Parochial School Students in Grades 7 through 12. New York, 1978.
4. New York State Division of Substance Abuse Services. Substance Use Among New York State Public and Private School Students in Grades 7 through 12. New York, 1984.
5. New York State Division of Substance Abuse Services. Drug Use in New York State A Report on the Nonmedical Use of Drugs Among the New York State Household Population New York, 1978.
6. New York State Division of Substance Abuse Services. Preliminary Report: Drug Use Among New York State's Household Population. New York, 1981
7 New York State Division of Substance Abuse Services. Drug Use Among College Students in New York State. New York, 1981.
8 Frank, B., Schmeidler, J., Johnson, B., and Lipton, D.S. Seeking Truth in Heroin Indicators: The Case of New York City. Drug Alcohol Depen, 3, 345–358, 1978.
9. Pihl, R.O., Marinier, R., Lepp, J., and Drake, H. Psychotropic Drug Use by Women: Characteristics of High Consumers. Int. J. Addict. 17(2), 259–269, 1982.
10. Verbrugge. L.M Sex Differences in Legal Drug Use. J Soc Iss., 38(2), 59–76, 1982.
11. Stimson, G. Women in a doctored world. New Soc. 32, 265–267, 1975.

The Effect
of Multiple Family Therapy
on Addict Family Functioning:
A Pilot Study

Thomas R. Kosten, MD
Izola Hogan, RN
Behnaz Jalali, MD
John Steidl, MSW
Herbert D. Kleber, MD

ABSTRACT. Family therapy may help addicts remain drug abstinent by improving family functioning. In a outpatient pilot study eight addict families were evaluated before and after 16 weeks of multiple family therapy (MFT), while the addict was maintained on naltrexone, an opiate antagonist. The Beavers Timberlawn Family Assessment was used to rate videotapes on problem solving, family structure, individual autonomy, and affect. The 8 families showed significant improvement in global functioning, problem solving, structure, and autonomy, but not in affect. One addict relapsed during the 10 month follow up, and his was the only family that functioned worse at follow up. We concluded that MFT can help addict families progress from chaotic interactions to more stable family structures and from rigid to more flexible family functioning. This improvement in family functioning may be associated with ex-addicts remaining abstinent.

The authors are affiliated with the Yale University School of Medicine, Department of Psychiatry, Connecticut Mental Health Center, Addiction Prevention Treatment Foundation in the following capacities: Thomas R. Kosten as Assistant Professor, Izola Hogan as Head Nurse, Behnaz Jalali and John Steidl as Associate Clinical Professors, and Herbert Kleber as Professor. Please address reprint requests to T.R. Kosten, MD, APT Foundation, 904 Howard Avenue—Suite 1A, New Haven, CT 06510.

INTRODUCTION

In a review of the effectiveness of family therapy across settings and diagnostic groups DeWitt[1] concluded that family therapy was at least as good as, if not superior to, other methods of psychiatric treatment. In support of this conclusion several studies with opiate addicts have demonstrated that effectiveness of family therapy in maintaining drug abstinence.[2-5] Furthermore, in a recent book on the family therapy of addicts Stanton and Todd[3] concluded that specific changes in family behavior are associated with drug abstinence. Videotapes of their therapy sessions were reviewed and detailed case histories showed specific family changes.

These findings are most important to the field of substance abuse and need further testing through controlled trials. However, as a first step, assessment instruments for making systematic comparisons of family functioning before and after treatment need to be tested with addict families. If an instrument can detect significant changes between the pre- and post-treatment assessments, then the instrument would have demonstrated satisfactory sensitivity to the degree of change that might be expected with treatment of these families. Furthermore, significant improvement in these assessments would support using this instrument for more extensive controlled clinical trials of addict family treatment. Because changes over time may be due to non-specific effects of participation in any treatment or even repeated assessments, definitive conclusions about the efficacy of family treatment in addicts cannot be drawn from this type of pilot work. However, pilot work is needed to guide decisions about selecting appropriate assessment instruments for evaluations of established treatment programs, as well as for designing controlled studies.

The current study focused on addict families who completed 16 sessions of outpatient weekly multiple family therapy (MFT), a relatively novel approach for outpatient opioid addicts. The purpose of this pilot study was to compare the functioning of these families before starting multiple family therapy to their level of functioning after completing it. As a clinical study, we were also interested in whether MFT might improve specific areas of family functioning and not affect other areas. Thus, several areas of family functioning were assessed using an instrument new to the drug abuse field—the Beavers Timberlawn Family Assessment Guide.[6] Using this Guide subscales were developed to measure four areas: problem solving, family structure, individual autonomy and affective expression.

METHODS

Sample

Eight opiate addicts and their families were evaluated both before family treatment and four to 16 months (10 ± 4 months) after the addict entered our opiate antagonist treatment program. The addicts had a mean age of 26, one was female and all were white. Five were treated with their parents and five with their spouse. Two had both their parents and spouse with them in treatment. No other family members in the household were current substance abusers, although two addicts had brothers who had histories of substance abuse. Two of the unmarried addicts were unemployed, but obtained training or employment by the end of the family therapy. These two addicts also did not complete high school. Two other addicts had had some college courses. The mean duration of opiate abuse was 4.9 years.

Treatment Setting

Naltrexone is an orally effective opioid antagonist usually given three times per week to drug-free ex-addicts. The use of naltrexone and the details of our treatment program have been described previously.[2,7,8,9] Addicts took naltrexone for about six months and were then followed with at least weekly random urine monitoring for six to 18 months. Within this program weekly family therapy occurred in open multiple family groups with a psychiatrist as co-therapist. Families participated for 16 weeks. Based on the work of Bowen[10] the family groups focused on family bonds and expectations and multi-generational patterns using a genogram. When clinically appropriate, a structural strategic approach was also utilized as described by Stanton and Todd.[3] The objectives of the family treatment were: (1) education and immediate problem solving, (2) helping addicts to disengage from enmeshed families or helping disengaged families to reestablish ties and helping parents to establish appropriate generational boundaries, (3) supporting family limit setting on the addict without open conflict, (4) supporting the addict's employment, education and assumption of responsibility. In addition to the family groups, problem oriented individual counseling was available for the ex-addict from the co-therapist who was not a psychiatrist. This individual counseling was generally not utilized during the family treatment.

Family Assessment

The addicts and their families were asked to participate in a 30 minute videotaped family interview within four weeks of the addict first coming to the naltrexone program. The family then completed 16 weeks of family therapy, and a second interview was videotaped one to 12 months after completing the family therapy.

Each family was seated in a room with a video camera that was operated by remote control. They were given an audiotape recorder with recorded instructions that asked them to complete the following five tasks derived from Minuchin's Wiltwyck project:[11] (1) plan a limited choice menu together; (2) identify the various roles family members fulfill, such as troublemaker, crybaby, etc; (3) discuss in detail a recent argument; (4) offer positive and negative feedback to each member of the family; (5) discuss changes experienced since the family has known about the drug abuse. The videotaped interview was later reviewed by two experienced family therapists (B.J. and J.H.S.) neither of whom were involved in the drug treatment.

Four general areas of family functioning corresponding to our family treatment objectives were assessed using the Beavers Timberlawn Family Assessment Guide.[6] The four areas were rated on a nine point family health pathology continuum and included problem solving, family structure, affect and individual autonomy. The structure area was assessed by combining the leadership and control, the parental coalition, the individual closeness and boundaries, and the generational boundaries items of the Beavers Timberlawn Guide. The affect area was assessed by combining the expression of thoughts and feelings, the mood and tone of family interactions, the empathy and the open conflict items. The autonomy area was assessed by combining the clarity of self concept, responsibility, invasiveness and openness to feedback items. Problem solving was a single item. These combinations of items followed the theoretical framework from which the Beavers Timberlawn Guide was developed.[6] High scores (7 to 9) indicated flexible and effective functioning on that dimension of family life, intermediate scores (4 to 6) indicated rigid but reasonably effective functioning on that dimension, and low scores (1 to 3) indicated chaotic and ineffective functioning on that dimension. A global family assessment was also made using this scoring system. Interrater reliability on these dimensions ranged from 0.66 to 0.90 with the median intraclass correlation being 0.80, indicating excellent interrater agreement.

Data Analysis

Scores for the families were computed by using the average of the two independent raters' scores on the nine point ordinal scales. This averaging yielded scores that often included fractional values for an individual family (e.g., 3.5 rather than 3 or 4). Because of the ordinal scaling of the Beavers Guide and the small number of subjects, the difference between the initial and follow-up scores for the eight families were compared using the non-parametric Wilcoxon Signed Rank Test for paired comparisons.[12] Because only one instrument was used with a single global rating and four subscales, corrections for multiple comparisons was unnecessary. To estimate the interrelationship between the four subscales and to relate these scales to age and length of follow-up Spearman rank correlations were used.

RESULTS

As a group the eight families significantly improved their family functioning following the family therapy. The initial global rating was at the low end of rigid family functioning

(4.5) reflecting poor negotiation during the simple Wiltwyck Tasks (i.e., the menu—Task 1) and an inability to complete the more complex tasks (i.e., offer positive and negative feedback—Task 4). At follow up these families improved to the upper end of rigid family functioning (5.8) reflecting their improved performance on the more complex Wiltwyck Tasks. They described rather than recreating a recent argument during the third Task and offered some realistic feedback to each other on the fourth Task. This improvement was statistically significant using Wilcoxon's T score for paired comparisons ($T = 3.5$, $n = 8$, $p < 0.05$). All of the families were at least in the midrange of functioning after treatment. For the individual families three showed substantial improvements in their global scores: 3 to 6, 5 to 7.5, 5 to 7, and four families had less improvment ranging from 0.5 to 1.5 points. One family became worse going from 6.5 to 5.5.

Since the global assessment demonstrated significant improvement, we investigated the four areas of family functioning (e.g., subscales) to identify specific changes related to the treatment. Problem solving showed the most significant improvement going from the low (4.0) to the high (5.9) midrange of functioning with improved negotiation and efficiency (Wilcoxon $T = 1$, $n = 8$, $p < 0.02$). Family structure improved into the high midrange of rigid structure with clear control and boundaries (5.1 to 6.3, Wilcoxon $T = 2$, $n = 8$, $p < 0.02$), and along with this stronger family structure, individual autonomy also increased (5.5 to 6.2, Wilcoxon $T = 4$, $n = 8$, $p < 0.05$). Family affect showed no significant change (5.1 to 5.8), although the conflict item of this scale indicated a reduction in the frequency of fighting (3.6 to 4.8, Wilcoxon $T = 3$, $n = 8$, $p < 0.05$). This reduction in fighting came at the expense of one family member now dictating rules and winning fights.

These four areas of family functioning (subscales) were relatively independent of each other. To estimate the interrelationship of these four subscales, seven Spearman correlations were computed, and only problem solving and family structure were significantly associated ($r = 0.79$, $p < 0.05$). The other areas had an average shared variance of 35% suggesting that these four subscales were not simply all measuring the same type of change among the eight families.

The treatment improvements were not associated with particular demographic factors in the sample or with the duration of follow up. Age was not significantly correlated with the change in global functioning or with any of the four subscales. The one family which included a female addict was among the three families showing the most improvement, but excluding this family did not change the overall results. All families had completed the full 16 weeks of family therapy and were reinterviewed one to 12 months after completing family therapy. The length of time between the initial and follow up interviews did not correlate with any changes in family functioning. Between the two interviews only one addict had returned to drug abuse, and the follow up interview had occurred when he returned to the drug treatment program. This was the only family to show a worsening in family functioning and no improvement in family problem solving.

DISCUSSION

Following 16 weeks of multiple family therapy in an outpatient opiate antagonist program eight addicts and their families demonstrated significant improvements in family functioning. Three areas of family functioning were significant contributors to this global improvement: problem solving, family structure and individual autonomy within the family. The family affect scale including family mood, empathy and the open expression of feelings did not show improvement, although the item on open conflict indicated that these families went from constant unresolved fights to intermittent fights that one family member usually won. Although family problems were hardly ever resolved by compromise and flexible negotiation, the family treatment was followed by significant improvement in family problem solving.

Because there is currently a growing interest in work with addicts and their families,[3,5] the treatment context and any differences in the response to treatment among the individual families are clearly important issues in attempting to apply these findings to ongoing treatment programs. Two central elements of the treatment context were the use of naltrexone in an outpatient program and the use of multiple family therapy

(MFT) rather than individual family therapy. Naltrexone, an opioid antagonist, is soon to be released for general use and may greatly improve the possibility for successful drug free outpatient treatment of addicts, if strategies can be developed to insure that addicts take it regularly.[7] Family support can make a major contribution to insuring this compliance with naltrexone,[2,9] and family therapy should be strongly considered to facilitate this support. Family therapy can also facilitate opioid detoxification. Stanton et al.[3] have elegantly applied family therapy to the detoxification of methadone maintained ex-addicts. Following detoxification family therapy might be continued with these ex-addicts while taking naltrexone to decrease the likelihood of relapse.[13] Family therapy has also been used with residential treatment and may be continued in conjunction with naltrexone in the outside community.[4,5] Thus, naltrexone treatment may have a substantial role to play in outpatient family treatment of addicts, either for addicts off the street, as in the present study, or for addicts in transition following family interventions that begin within methadone maintenance or residential treatment programs.

The second element of the treatment context was multiple family therapy (MFT). Addicts have been treated using MFT in previous clinical studies,[4,5] but the one randomized, controlled study in addicts used individual family therapy.[3] That controlled study utilized many techniques of structural family therapy that were an integral part of our MFT, and most of the strategies of that type of family therapy can be adapted to work in a MFT group. Furthermore, the emotional support of the group can often help enmeshed parents to separate from the addict, and this has been considered a central family problem in addiction.[3] It is also important to emphasize that MFT must be individualized for each family and for different groups and that psychotherapy, not simply didactic presentations, were the content of the MFT. Thus, the distinction between MFT and individual family therapy may be small for the actual conduct of this type of family therapy in addict families. Finally, in selecting individual or multiple family therapy available resources may need consideration, and MFT is clearly the most cost effective.

A second issue was individual differences among the families in their response to MFT. When the individual families were studied in detail, most of them showed substantially improved problem solving abilities. All three families who were in the more severe and chaotic range of dysfunction (scores from 1-3) at the start of treatment improved and moved into the more structured albeit midrange of functioning. The largest improvement was evident for the individual autonomy and problem solving areas. In other words, these very poorly functioning families learned how to make their individual thoughts and feelings about issues clearer and to listen more to each other. They then appeared to use this capacity for more efficient problem solving.

Five families were more rigidly structured before starting family treatment (scores from 4–6). The two families in the lower end of this mid-range (mean = 4.5) showed only modest improvement and remained within the mid-range after treatment. The family structure of these two families shifted from dictatorial leadership to more negotiated decision making on the Wiltwyck tasks, but problem solving did not substantially improve. Because problem solving involved both efficiency and negotiation, this lack of improved problem solving even with better negotiation could be easily understood. With more negotiation each of the tasks took longer and seemed less efficient. Nevertheless, a real improvement in the way problems were approached has occurred, because of this negotiation. The next two higher scoring families began in the midrange and moved into the upper range. They demonstrated more adaptive functioning in every area except family affect and showed substantial improvement in family problem solving. Finally, the family with the highest initial level of functioning (6.5 global rating) was the only family to show deterioration in functioning. The addict in this family relapsed to drug abuse, and when he returned to treatment, the reevaluation was done. Interestingly, only their problem solving had not deteriorated. Thus, these mid-range families demonstrated substantial variation in their response to family treatment, including some deterioration in a family whose son had relapsed to drug abuse during the several months since they had finished the family treatment.

In this treatment study we found that task oriented, executive functions showed the most change with family therapy. The areas of improvement and their intercorrelations suggested that these families generally progressed from somewhat chaotic, constantly fighting families who were unable to effectively solve problems to rigid but relatively peaceful families who resolved problems by authoritarian decision making. This improved executive functioning and reduced family conflict were associated with the addict remaining drug free in all except one case.

The association between executive functioning and drug abstinence seemed to contradict previous work in which executive family functions were not strongly associated with the addict remaining drug free.[9,16] In these prognostic studies baseline family functioning was used to predict relapse to drug abuse. The mood and tone of family interactions and the family's inability to communicate with each other, including such simple communications as the family openly admitting that the drug abuse had occurred, were associated with relapse to drug abuse.[9,16] This previous work suggested that family affect and communications were the most likely target areas for an intervention that would reduce drug abuse relapse. Since these affect and communications areas showed little change during this current intervention study, the ultimate effectiveness of this intervention on subsequent drug abuse must be considered.

An interactional, structural model of family change suggests that change in family structure will eventually impact on other areas of functioning. If the family is conceptualized as an open system with change resulting from circular rather than linear processes, then the improvement that we demonstrated in executive functions should lead to eventual improvement in other areas of the family system including affect and communications.[14] This family system change would then be associated with a reduced rate of relapse to drug abuse. A larger sample with a 12 to 18 month follow up for every family is needed to address these issues of specific change and its generalization over time, and these issues should probably be addressed in the context of a randomized clinical trial of family therapy.

Another important association in the prognostic studies was that between family conflict and relapse to drug abuse.[16] In the current study family conflict was the only item in the affect area that significantly decreased. The studies of expressed emotion in the families of schizophrenic patients have suggested that family conflicts are associated with relapse into psychosis,[15] and family interventions to reduce this expressed emotion might reduce relapse. A similar relationship between family conflict and drug abuse relapse may exist for addicts and their families. Therefore, family interventions such as ours that reduce these conflicts are potentially very useful. Futher study of this issue is needed, but an interesting parallel can be deduced between the studies of expressed emotion and our findings.

Our conclusions are limited by several features of this study. First, the sample was self selected for a special treatment program, naltrexone, and only included those addicts and their families who completed the 16 week family treatment program. Second, the sample included only white addicts. These limitations suggest that any generalization to other addict groups must be cautious. Third, as a treatment study this is clearly only a pilot for a larger randomized design, and in future studies appropriate controls need to be provided for merely getting the family together over several months. The most important finding may be the sensitivity of our family assessment to changes that seemed to be associated with drug abstinence. Future treatment studies should consider using the Beavers Timberlawn Family Assessment Guide for assessing change.

REFERENCES

1. Dewitt KN. The effectiveness of family therapy. Arch Gen Psychiatry. 1978. 35: 549–561.

2. Anton RF, Hogan I. Jalali B, Riordan CE, Kleber HD. Multiple family therapy and naltrexone in the treatment of opioid dependence. Drug Alcohol Depend. 1981. 8: 157–168

3. Stanton MD, Todd TC, et al. *The Family Therapy of Drug Abuse and Addiction. 1982. New York, Guilford Press.*

4. Hendricks WJ. Use of multifamily counseling groups in the treatment of male narcotic addicts. Int J Group Psychotherapy. 1971. 21: 84–90

5. Kaufman E, Kaufman P (eds). *Family Therapy of Drug and Alcohol Abusers.* 1979 New York, Halstead Press.

6. Lewis JM, Beavers WR, Gossett JT, et al. *No Single Thread: Psychological Health in Family Systems.* 1976. New York, Brunner Mazel Inc. pp. 46–98.

7. Kosten TR, Kleber HD. Strategies to improve compliance with narcotic antagonists. Amer J Drug Alcohol Abuse. 1984. 10: 249–266.

8. Kosten TR, Jalali B, Kleber HD. Complementary marital roles in male heroin addicts. Amer J Drug Alcohol Abuse. 1982. 9: 155–169

9. Kosten TR, Jalali B, Hogan I, Kleber HD. Family denial as a prognostic factor in opiate addict treatment outcome. J Nervous Mental Dis. 1983. 171: 606–611.

10. Bowen M. Multiple family therapy. In Guerin P (ed) *Family Therapy: Theory and Practice.* 1976 New York, Gardner Press. pp. 388–404.

11. Minuchin S, Montalvo B, Guerney B, et al. *Families of the Slums. An Exploration of Their Structure and Treatment.* 1967. New York, Basic Books. Chap. 7.

12. Blalock HM Jr. Social Statistics. 2nd Edition. New York, McGraw-Hill Book Co. 1979. pp. 269–273 and Appendix Table H.

13. Kosten TR, Astrachan BM, Riordan CE, Kleber HD. The organization of a methadone maintenance program J Drug Issues. 1982. Fall: 333–342.

14. Minuchin S, Fishman HC. *Family Therapy Techniques.* 1982. Cambridge, Mass., Harvard University Press.

15. Brown GW, Birley JLT, Wing JK. Influence of family life on the course of schizophrenic disorders: a replication. Brit J Psychiatry. 1972 121: 241–258.

16. Kosten TR, Jalali B, Steidl JS, Kleber HD. Relationship of marital structure and interactions to opiate abuse relapses (in press). Amer J Drug Alcohol Abuse.

Adolescents' Substance Use: Impact of Ethnicity, Income, and Availability

Ebrahim Maddahian, PhD
Michael D. Newcomb, PhD
P. M. Bentler, PhD

ABSTRACT. This study examines ethnic differences in reported use of cigarettes, alcohol, cannabis, hard drugs, and non-prescription medications among a sample of adolescents and attempts to explain these differences in terms of income, ease of acquisition, and availability from friends. Data were obtained from 847 students three times over a five-year period. Results indicate consistent and significant differences among ethnic groups substance use at all three points in time. It was hypothesized that ethnic groups have differential access to substances and economic resources to purchase various drugs. To test these hypotheses, availability from friends, perceived ease of acquisition, income from earnings and gifts/allowances, and initial substance use were examined across ethnic groups and then used as covariates of the substance differences. A split-plot repeated measures design with covariates was used to compare changes in substance use across time and between ethnic groups. Earned income made a significant impact on explaining the ethnic differences for cigarette, alcohol, and given income on cannabis consumption. Adding community variables such as availability from friends, ease of acquisition, and initial drug use not only eliminates the effects of income variables on drug use, but in most cases, the ethnic differences among adolescents as well.

Drs. Maddahian, Newcomb, and Bentler are with the Department of Psychology, University of California, Los Angeles, CA. This research was partially supported by Grant Number DA 01070 from the U.S. Public Health Service. The production assistance of Julie Speckart is gratefully acknowledged. Address correspondence to Dr. Ebrahim Maddahian, Department of Psychology, U.C.L.A., Los Angeles, California, 90024.

63

INTRODUCTION

For quite some time there has been an awareness among professionals and the general population that substance use is both a pervasive and significant community problem, particularly among young and impressionable adolescents.[1-3] Nearly everyone can recall an adverse social or personal event that could be linked to the use of alcohol or other drugs. Such unpleasant events as accidents, violence, dropping out of school, and addiction are among the most serious drug related problems. Concern for preventing such tragedies leads one to consider causal influences for the use of drugs among the young. Three possible antecedent conditions that may have an impact on choosing to use certain drug substances are the social/psychological influences associated with belonging to a particular ethnic group, differential income levels necessary for the acquisition of drugs, and different levels of availability of drug substances in the individual's environment.

Although several studies have noted differences in rates of licit and illicit substance use across various ethnic groups [4-10] it remains unclear how early these differences occur and whether they are consistent or stable over time. For example, in a recent survey of substance use among high school students, it was found that white students use more drugs than students from other ethnic groups, except American Indians who reported unusually high rates of use.[11]

One plausible explanation for finding different rates of substance use across ethnic groups (assuming equal availability) is that certain ethnic groups may have more money to spend on drugs than others. In other words, perhaps the reason that white students reported greater use of drugs than most other ethnic groups is due to white students having more money and thus able to purchase drugs at their pleasure. Among adult populations, several studies have noted associations between drug use and income related variables such as salary and employment status.[12-16] However, contrary to Kandel's[14] observation that the unemployed men have the highest rate of drug use, Bachman et al.[13] found that unemployed men actually used less marijuana and other illicit drugs than when they were in high school. One possible explanation is that these men have less money to purchase drugs when they are not employed. However, very little research has examined the relationship between substance use and income among adolescents, perhaps because teenagers are not typically employed full-time or have a regular income.

One exception to this omission is a recent study by Mills and Noyes.[17] They found that the amount of available spending money is a significant predictor of substance use (e.g., alcohol, marijuana, cocaine) among 8th, 10th, and 12th grade high school students. Udell, Smith, and Edwards[18] also found that children from higher socio-economic status reported greater use of marijuana than lower class groups, again, implying that economic resources may moderate the degree of drug use among adolescents.

A second plausible explanation is that different levels of access to substances may exist among adolescents from different ethnicities. Bauman,[19] Kandel, Kessler, and Margulies,[20] and Rawbow et al.[16] particularly emphasize the relationship between substance use and its availability in the community. Although there have been several studies that have examined substance use and abuse among minority groups,[6, 21-24] the majority of drug research has focused largely on middle-class white population. This study examines reported drug use among Hispanic, Black, Asian, and White adolescents at three points in time over a five-year span, and attempts to account for the ethnic differences by controlling for earned income (salaries), given income (allowances/gifts), availability of substance through friends, ease of substance acquisition, and initial substance use.

METHOD

Subjects

Participants in this study are 847 students, originally in 7th, 8th, and 9th grades located at 11 schools in the Los Angeles County. During the first year of data collection (1976), 1634 adolescents participated in a longitudinal study of adolescents and provided complete sets of data. Although a second wave of data was obtained in 1977, it will not be included in this report due to a limited number of drug use items and other data. At the third wave of data collection (4th year, 1979), 1068 students participated, while during the fourth phase of the longitudinal study (5th year, 1980) 896 students completed the questionnaires.

A breakdown of the original sample (N = 1634) by grade, sex and ethnicity is given by Huba, Wingard, & Bentler.[25] Of the 847 selected subjects for this study, 110 (13.0%) are Hispanic, 135 (15.3%) Black, 65 (7.7%) Asian, and 542 (64.0%) White. About one-third of the sample (277) were male and slightly more than two-thirds (570) were female. Table 1 presents the sample by ethnicity breakdown at three data points over the 5 year period of study, from 1976 to 1980. This study uses 847 students who completed questionnaires at all three waves of data collection, first, fourth and fifth years, which represents 52% of the original sample.

Drug Use Assessment

In the first year of the study, each subject completed a questionnaire that assessed the rate of use for 13 different drug substances. Lifetime frequency-of-use data were collected for cigarettes, beer, wine, liquor, cocaine, tranquilizers, non-prescription medication used to get high, heroin and other opiates, marijuana, hashish, inhalants, hallucinogens, and amphetamines. Subject responses were recorded on anchored five-point scales with the following response catego-

Table 1

Cross-Tabulation of Sample by Ethnicity and Study Phase

Phase	Hispanic	Black	Asian	White	Total
Phase I (1st year)	242 (14.8)*	385 (23.6)	85 (5.2)	922 (56.4)	1634 (100)
Phase III (4th year)	155 (9.5)	181 (11.1)	73 (4.5)	659 (40.3)	1068 (65.4)
Phase IV (5th year)	117 (7.1)	152 (9.3)	67 (4.1)	560 (34.3)	896 (54.8)
Study Sample	110 (6.7)	135 (8.3)	65 (4.0)	542 (33.2)	847 (51.8)

* Parentheses contain the percent of the total original sample (N = 1634).

ries and scale values: (1) never tried; (2) only once; (3) a few times; (4) many times; and (5) regularly.

During the third and fourth phases of the study (year 4 and 5), the original 13-item drug questionnaire was expanded to include 26 different drugs. Subjects were asked to rate their frequency of drug use during the past six months on an anchored rating scale ranging from 1 to 7 with categories coded (1) never; (2) once or twice; (3) a few times; (4) once a month; (5) once a week; (6) once a day; and (7) more than once a day.

Income Variables

Fifth year participants were asked to indicate their income (salaries and wages) on a scale of 1 to 7 in July 1979, October 1979, and January of 1980, coded as (1) none; (2) $1 to $50; (3) $51 to $100; (4) $101 to $200; (5) $201 to $300; (6) $301 to $500; and (7) more than $500. They also were asked to indicate the amount of money they received in allowances or gifts on a seven-point scale that ranged from (1) none to (7) $50 or more during the same three months. The average of the three salary and wage items were used as indication of earned income, while the average of the three allowance and gift items was called given income.

Environmental Variables

Three sets of variables are used as indicators of adolescent's living environment, availability from friends, ease of substance acquisition, and initial substance use. Availability of substances from friends (availability from friends) was measured by a general question asking "How many of your friends have given you _____?" and rated for cigarettes, alcohol (beer/wine, or liquor), marijuana, narcotics (cocaine or heroin), and PCP on a scale of (1) none, (2) some, (3) many, (4) most, and (5) all. These items were utilized in the fourth and fifth years of the study. Alcohol availability from friends is the average of two questions related to beer/wine and liquor. Hard drug availability is the average of narcotics (cocaine or heroin) and PCP availability.

Perceived ease of substance acquisition (ease of acquisition) was measured by asking the participants "How hard or easy would it be to get _____?" filled in by cigarettes, alcohol (beer, wine, and liquor), cannabis (marijuana or hashish) and other drugs (e.g., uppers, downers, heroin, PCP and LSD). Responses were anchored on a 5-point scale of (1) very hard to (5) very easy. Alcohol ease of acquisition was the average of responses for beer, wine, and liquor.

Initial substance use variables were used as indicators of early drug involvement. These variables are initial cigarettes use, alcohol consumption, cannabis use, non-prescription medication and hard drug use. When these variables were assessed (year 1), the participants were in the seventh, eighth, and ninth grades, with an average age of 13.1 and presumably still under the influence of their family. Initial cigarettes use is composed of only one item. The alcohol scale is the average of the sum of beer, wine and liquor consumption. Initial cannabis use is the average use of marijuana and hashish. Initial non-prescription medication use was represented by only one item, and initial hard drug use is the average use of 6 items including cocaine, downers, narcotics, inhalants, hallucinogens, and uppers. Because of rating scale discrepancies between year 1 and years 4 or 5, first year scales are generally used only as covariates.

Some Methodological Considerations

One difficulty in comparing substance means over time arises from the large number of substances assessed in the fourth and fifth year of the study. Comparable scales of the items were constructed based on factor analyses,[26] the nature of the substances, and previous drug use research.[27] These constructed scales are: cigarettes; cannabis; alcohol; non-prescription medicines; and hard drugs. Cigarette use is composed of only one item. Cannabis use is the average of marijuana and hashish use. The alcohol scale is the average of the sum of beer, wine and liquor use. The non-prescription medication scale was represented by four items in the fourth and fifth years: nonprescription sleeping pills, stimulants, cough medicines, and cold/allergy medicines. The hard drugs scale was an average of 14 items in the fourth and fifth year (e.g., barbiturates, LSD, amphetamines, heroin, cocaine,

PCP). Drinking coffee or tea and use of amyl nitrate were excluded from the scales because no significant and clear pattern of loadings was found for these items in the factor analyses. These fourth and fifth year substance scales were used as dependent variables for the study analyses.

As with all longitudinal studies, our sample has been affected by attrition. An extensive series of analyses were conducted to determine the impact of subject dropout. There was greater attrition among Black and Hispanic groups than the White and Asian groups. However, the pattern of drug use did not dramatically change because of this differential loss of participants. In other words, the rank ordering of substance use levels did not change due to attrition effects. As a result, we feel confident that the results presented in this paper arise from the substantive nature of the inquiry and are not an artifact of attrition.

Analyses

Three sets of analyses were executed to examine the pattern of substance use among adolescents from different ethnic backgrounds. One-way analyses of variance were used to compare the means of variables for possible ethnic differences, along with pairwise comparison among group means where significant, using the Bonferroni method to adjust p-values for multiple post hoc comparisons. A repeated measures design was used to detect changes in the pattern of substance use over time for each ethnic group. Finally, covariance split-plot design with repeated measures was used to test the change in drug use pattern over time among the Hispanic, Black, Asian and White samples, while controlling for the effects of earned and given income, availability from friends, ease of acquisition, and initial use of substances. In this design, ethnicity is a between factor, year represents a within factor, and income, initial use and ease of acquisition as fixed covariates and availability from friends is a changing covariate. Changing covariates are paired with the dependent variables. that is, the first covariate is nested as covariate for the first level of the within factor and second covariate for the second level.[28, 29]

RESULTS

Substance Use Pattern

T-tests were used to determine whether there were sex differences on the five substance use scales. Female adolescents showed higher levels of cigarette smoking than males at all three time points. No significant difference was found between males and females on alcohol consumption or marijuana use. Females also reported a higher level of use for non-prescription medicines in the last two years of the study. No significant difference was found between males and females on hard drugs except for the fifth year, where the female mean was slightly higher than the male mean (1.09 vs. 1.07).

Although gender is a significant predictor of use for some substances, none of the intraclass correlations between sex and substance use was higher than .01. In that gender accounts for less than 1% of the substance use variance, the sexes were combined for the subsequent analyses.

Two sets of analyses were conducted to test whether (a) there are significant differences for substance use among the four ethnic groups; and (b) there are significant changes in substance use across time for each group over the last two-year period of the study. Table 2 presents the results of the between group analyses for all five substance use scales as well as pairwise comparison among group means.

It was found that significant differences exist among adolescents' initial substance use on cigarette smoking, alcohol consumption, cannabis use, and the use of non-prescription medications. The top portion of Table 2 presents the overall F-values as well as pairwise comparisons among means of initial substance use for each ethnic group. Asian adolescents' initial level of cigarette smoking is lower than other groups. Blacks' initial level of alcohol consumption is lower than Whites and Hispanics. Cannabis use among Whites is significantly greater than Asians, while use of nonprescription medications is greater for Whites than Blacks. No significant differences were found among ethnic groups for initial hard drug use.

Initial substance use data are responses given for life-time use, while the substance use data in subsequent years (fourth and fifth year) are limited to a retrospective period of 6

Table 2

Summary of the one-way analysis of substance use scales (N = 847)

Substance use Scale	Year	Hispanic	Black	Asian	White	F^w-value
Initial use						
Cigarettes	1	2.36[a]	2.42[b]	1.68[a,b,c]	2 18[c]	9.43***
Alcohol	1	2.33[b]	2.00[a,b]	2.10	2.43[a]	9.72***
Cannabis	1	1.35	1 29	1 14[a]	1 39[a]	4.84**
Non-prescription drugs	1	1.19	1.07[a]	1.25	1.25[a]	5.42***
Hard drug	1	1.10	1 08	1.08	1 09	0.16
Fourth and Fifth Year Substance Use						
Cigarettes	4	2.22	2 56[a]	1.72[a,b]	2.28[b]	4.00**
	5	2.41	2 74[a]	1.91[a]	2.43	2.73*
Across time F-ratio		1 34	1.28	2.22	4 52*	
Alcohol	4	2 47[a]	1 80[a,b]	2.01[c]	2.53[b,c]	18.01***
	5	2.54[a]	1 97[a,b]	2.17[c]	2 65[b,c]	13.69***
Across time F-ratio		0 66	3 76	1.61	6.50*	
Cannabis	4	1.87[a]	1.60[b]	1 39[a,c]	2.06[b,c]	12.42***
	5	2.03[a]	1.84	1.52[a,b]	2.14[b]	7.46***
Across time F-ratio		2.45	8.82**	3 67	3.41	
Non-prescription drugs	4	1.61	1.48	1 67	1.55	1.55
	5	1.44	1 34	1.54	1.43	2.21
Across time F-ratio		8 07**	6.14**	2.68	22.27***	
Hard drugs	4	1 10[a]	1 02[a,b]	1 06	1.11[b]	15.99***
	5	1 10[a]	1.02[a,b]	1.06	1.14[b]	25.53***
Across time F-ratio		0 01	0 07	0.14	8.24**	

F^w Welch F-ratio assuming unequal group variances. Similar letters indicate significant differences within a row.

* $p \leq$ 05, ** $p \leq$ .01, *** $p \leq$ 001.

months. Due to this time frame difference and also rating scale differences, no comparisons were made between initial substance use scales and fourth or fifth year substance use scales. First year substance use data are utilized as covariates in latter analyses.

During the last two years of the study, there are significant differences across ethnic groups for all substance scales except for the non-prescription medication (see bottom portion of

Table 2). Although the overall F-ratios are significant for cigarette smoking, there is some indication that these differences may diminish over time. While in the fourth year there is a significant difference between both Blacks and Whites versus Asians for cigarette smoking, at the fifth year the difference remains significant only between Blacks and Asians.

Although the level of alcohol consumption is consistently different among most ethnic groups at both time periods, there is no significant difference between Hispanics and Whites. Alcohol consumption for Whites is consistently higher than Blacks and Asians, while Hispanics report greater use than Blacks. For cannabis use, there is also a significant overall difference by ethnicity at both time periods. Whites' and Hispanics' cannabis use is consistently higher than Asians'. The difference between cannabis use for Whites and Blacks noted in year four decreases by year five.

While there is no significant difference among the means of the nonprescription medication scale across ethnic groups, there is a consistent difference among the ethnic groups on hard drug use for both year four and five. The means of Whites and Hispanics are consistently higher than Blacks.

Across time analyses showed that there are significant increases in the level of cigarette smoking (F = 4.52, p < .05), alcohol consumption (F = 6.50, p < .05), and hard drugs use (F = 8.42, p < .01) for White students. However, their level of nonprescription drug use significantly decreases (F = 22.27, p < .001) from year 4 to 5. As indicated in Table 2, there is no significant change in the pattern of drug use over time for Asian adolescents. Blacks' level of cannabis use significantly increases (F = 8.82, p < .01) over time while their level of nonprescription medication use decreases (F = 6.14, p < .01). For the Hispanic group, there is only a significant decrease in the level of nonprescription drug use over time.

Ethnic Differences on Income, Availability from Friends, and Ease of Acquisition.

Income Differences. As indicated in the top part of Table 3, there is a significant difference among ethnic groups on both earned income (salaries and wages) and given income (allowances and gifts). Specifically, the mean of earned income for

Table 3

Summary of the mean comparisons of other study variables (N = 847)

Covariate	Year	Ethnicity				F^w-value
		Hispanic	Black	Asian	White	
Income:						
Earned income (salaries)	5	3.03	2.90[a]	3.56	3.56[a]	6.62***
Given income (allowances)	5	4.10	4.56[a,b]	3.72[a]	3.67[b]	7.99***
Substance availability.						
Friends give Cigarettes	4	1.67[a]	1.71[b]	1.29[a,b]	1.56	3.59*
Friends give Cigarettes	5	1.66	1.67	1.35	1.51	2.56
Friends give Marijuana	4	1.90[a]	1.62	1.40[a,b]	1.89[b]	9.84***
Friends give Marijuana	5	1.92[a,b]	1.51[b,c]	1.52[a,d]	1.90[c,d]	8.75***
Friends give Alcohol	4	2.08[a,b]	1 54[b,c]	1.62[a,d]	2.18[c,d]	26.68***
Friends give Alcohol	5	2.21[a,b]	1.60[b,c]	1 75[a,d]	2.30[c,d]	26.35***
Friends give Drugs	4	1.10[a]	1.03[a,b]	1.07	1.12[b]	11.14***
Friends give Drugs	5	1.20	1 08[b]	1.11[a]	1.22[a,b]	9.74***
Ease of substance acquisition						
Cigarettes	5	4 47	4.45	4.23[a]	4.67[a]	4.80**
Alcohol	5	4.09	3.81[b]	3.82[a]	4.26[a,b]	7.44***
Marijuana	5	3.86[a]	3 49	3.31[a,b]	3.82[b]	5.03**
Other drugs	5	3.18[a,b]	2.54[a,c]	2.63[b,d]	3.10[c,d]	8.37***

Welch F-ratio assuming unequal group variances.
Similar letters indicate significant differences within a row.

* p ≤ .05, ** p ≤ .01, *** p ≤ .001.

Whites is significantly higher than Blacks (3.56 vs. 2.90) while given income for Blacks is significantly higher than for both Whites and Asians (4.56 vs. 3.67 and 3.72).

Substance Availability Differences. Substance availability from friends in the 4th and 5th years of study were utilized as indicators of drug availability in the community for four major substances: cigarettes, cannabis, alcohol, and hard drugs. Except for fifth year given cigarettes by friends, all the F-values testing difference among ethnic groups are highly significant (middle part of Table 3). Blacks report the highest cigarette availability, Hispanics the greatest marijuana availability, and Whites the most alcohol and hard drugs availability.

Ease of Acquisition Differences. Overall significant differences as well as pairwise comparisions on the means of ease of acquisition variables are also presented in the bottom part of Table 3. In general, it is harder for Asian students to obtain most substances than Whites. It is harder for Blacks to obtain alcohol than Whites. No differences were found between White and Hispanic groups.

Covariate Analyses

To examine the effects of income, substance availability from friends, ease of substance acquisition, and initial substance use on the effects of ethnicity, three sets of analyses of covariance were conducted. In the first set of analyses, earned income and given income were controlled. In the second set of analyses substance availability from friends and ease of substance acquisition were introduced into the design in addition to the income variables. It should be noted that there are no corresponding variables for substance availability and ease of acquisition for non-prescription drugs. In the third set of covariate analyses initial substance use was added to the covariates already entered.

Income Effects. A split-plot repeated measure design using student's earned income and given income as covariates was used to control the income effects on substance use. The top portion of Table 4 presents a summary of the results of these analyses. It was found that students' earned income is a significant predictor of cigarette smoking and alcohol consumption. Earned income did not contribute to the prediction of cannabis, non-prescription drugs, and hard drug use. Given income contributes only to the prediction of non-prescription medication use. These variables, although significant predictors, did not explain all of the differences in ethnic substance use.

Availability and Ease of Acquisition Effects. Adding availability from friends and ease of acquisition of substances into the second design, substantially reduces the ethnic difference effect and also eliminates the effects of income variables (Table 4, second design). Substance availability from friends has a salient impact on all substance use at both between and within group levels. Ease of acquisition was also a significant predictor of all substances. No specific questions were asked for ease of acquisition or availability from friends on non-prescription drugs.

Initial Substance Use Effects. First year drug use data, clustered into five substance use scales noted above were utilized as measures of initial substance use and family influence.

Table 4

Summary of the F-values for 3 consecutive ANOVA splot-plot
repeated measure designs of substance use scales

Source of variance	Cigarettes	Alcohol	Cannabis	Non-prescription drugs	Hard Drugs
First design:					
Between groups:					
Ethnicity	2.92*	16.45***	7.55***	3.11*	8.12***
#Earned income (salaries)	4 51*	20.29***	1.81	0.97	0.39
#Given income (allowances)		0.17	3.47	0.35	4.65*
Within groups:					
Year	5.49*	7.21**	10.61**	25 42***	0.82
Year × Ethnicity	0.03	0.21	0.79	0.25	1.31
Second design:					
Between groups.					
Ethnicity	1 61	0.47	2.82*		1.34
#Earned income (salaries)	0 29	1 85	1.88		0.29
#Given income (allowances)	1.19	0.19	0.42		0 18
#Substance availability	1452.48***	957.97***	1589 94***		1242.14***
#Ease of substance acquisition	13 04***	15.49***	14.74***		5.25*
Within group:					
Year	7 00**	2.91	12.82***		3.32
Year × Ethnicity	0 03	0.42	1.96		1 05
#Substance availability	147.81***	137.13***	236.29***		369 85***
Third design:					
Between groups:					
Ethnicity	1.81	0.40	2.65*	2.76	1.39
#Earned income (salaries)	0.00	1.17	2.27	0.82	0.35
#Given income (allowances)	1 89	0.39	0 35	4 80*	0 14
#Substance availability	1120 38***	752 34***	1383 24***		1214 27***
#Ease of substance acquisition	6.13*	10.24**	13.52***		5.62*
#Initial use	60.36***	25.75***	7.35**	11.78***	8.94**
Within groups:					
Year	7.00**	2.91	12.82***	25.42	3.32
Year × Ethnicity	0 03	0.42	1.96	0.25	1.05
#Substance availability	147 81***	137.13	236.29***		369.85***

\# covariate

* $p \leq .05$, ** $p \leq 01$, *** $p \leq .001$.

Although initial substance use slightly reduces the effects of availability, it significantly contributes to the prediction of substance use in the later stage of adolescent drug use (Table 4, third design).

DISCUSSION

The analyses presented strongly indicate that there are consistent and significant differences in the pattern of substance use among continuing students from different ethnic backgrounds. The important questions are who is different from whom, on what kind of substance, and most importantly, why. It was found that while Blacks' cigarette smoking remains substantially and consistently higher than Asian adolescents', the difference between cigarette smoking of Whites and Asian adolescents decreases over time. Blacks show the highest level of smoking cigarettes followed by Whites (Table 2). One limitation of our sample is that it represents only one geographical area and thus generalizations to other areas must be made guardedly. However, our findings are very similar to other studies of ethnic differences on substance use.[2, 30-32]

White students consume significantly more alcohol than other ethnic groups, followed by Hispanics. The lowest level of alcohol use belongs to Black adolescents. White students also have the highest cannabis use followed by Hispanic students. Asians reported the lowest level of cannabis use over time. Although there was a trend for non-prescription drug use to be higher for Asian than other ethnic groups, no consistent and significant differences were found over the five-year duration of the study.

In terms of hard drugs, White adolescents again showed the highest level of use, followed by Hispanics. The lowest level of hard drug use is among Black students. Although Asians show a lower mean of hard drug use than Whites and Hispanics, the difference is not statistically different.

The implications of this study for Black students would be to emphasize the need for drug education and prevention focused mostly on cigarette smoking. White and Hispanic students need drug prevention and drug education centered on all the substances, especially alcohol, cannabis and hard drugs. Asian students showed high levels of non-prescription drug use and thus an emphasis should be in this direction. The pattern of substance use for Hispanics is very similar to Whites, while the Black and Asian patterns of substance use are different from each other and also from Whites and Hispanic groups.

Earned income is a significant predictor of cigarette smoking and alcohol consumption assuming equal availability. Given income is a significant predictor of nonprescription drug use. However, these effects drastically decrease when substance availability and ease of substance acquisition from friends are considered. One important point which should be highlighted here is that the consistent ethnic effects which remain strong even after introducing the income variables also decrease after the availability from friends and ease of acquisition of substances is controlled. These findings explain the importance of ethnic differences in terms of environmental factors. One implication from this might be that treatment programs for drug use and abuse should be community based and context oriented rather than merely individualized in treatment and separate from the social environment.

Finally, an early initiation into the drug culture is also a significant predictor of substance use. This issue has been noted previously in terms of modeling theory and mother's influence on their children's use of substances.[33] The results of this study clearly supports the influence of environment on substance use. Assuming that early use of substances is related to environmental conditions, family involvement in drug education and drug prevention programs must be considered.

REFERENCES

1. Coombs RH, Eckman TA, Swenson EW. The social and familial context of substance use among youth. In R. Faulkinberry (Ed.), *Drug: Problems of the 70's, solution for the 80's.* 1980.

2. Forster B. Upper middle class adolescent drug use: Patterns and factors. Advan Alcohol Substance Abuse. 1984; 4:27–36.

3. Johnston LD, O'Malley PM, Eveland LK. Drugs and delinquency: A search for causal connection. In Denise B. Kandel (Ed.), *Longitudinal research on drug use.* New York: John Wiley & Sons, 1978:137–156.

4. Ball JC, Chambers CD. Overview of the problem. In J. C. Ball & C. D. Chambers (Eds.), *The epidemiology of opiate addiction in the United States.* Springfield, Illinois: Charles C. Thomas, 1970.

5. Johnson BD. *Marijuana users and drug subcultures.* New York: Wiley, 1973.

6. Kaestner E, Rosen L, Appel P. Patterns of drug abuse: Relationships with ethnicity, sensation seeking and anxiety. J Consul Clin Psychol. 1977; 45:462–468.

7. Newcomb MD, Bentler PM. Ethnic comparisons of adolescent substance use: A longitudingal analysis. Presented at the Western Psychological Association, San Jose, California, 1985 April.

8. Newman RG, Cates M, Tytum A, Werbel B. Narcotic addiction in New York City: Trends from 1968 to mid 1972. Am J Drug Alcohol abuse. 1974; 1:53–66.

9. Single E, Kandel DB, Faust R. Patterns of multiple drug use in high school. J Health Soc Behavior. 1974; 15:344–357.

10. Wald PM, Hutt PB. The drug abuse survey project: Summary of findings, conclusions, and recommendations. In *Dealing with drug abuse: A report to the Ford Foundation.* New York: Praeger, 1972:3–61.

11. Skager R, Maddahian E. A survey of substance use and related factors among secondary school students in grades 7, 9, and 11 in the County of Orange. Fall 1983, *Report No. 224.* Center for Study of Evaluation, Graduate School of Education, University of California, Los Angeles, 1984.

12. Bachman JG, O'Malley PM, Johnston LD. Changes in drug use after high school as a function of role status and social environment. *Monitoring Future, Occasional Paper II,* Ann Arbor, MI: Institute for Social Research, 1981.

13. Bachman JG, O'Malley PM, Johnston LD. Drug use among adults: The impacts of role status and social environment. J Pers Soc Psychol. 1984; 47:629–645.

14. Kandel DB. Drug and drinking behavior among youth. Ann Rev Soc. 1980; 6:235–285.

15. Picov JS, Wells RH, Miranne AC. Marijuana use, occupational success values and materialistic orientations of university students: A research note. Adol. 1980; 15:529–534.

16. Rawbow J, Schwartz C, Stevens S, Watts RK. Social psychological dimensions of alcohol availability: The relationship of perceived social obligations, price considerations, and energy expended to the frequency, amount, and type of alcoholic beverage consumed. Int J Addict. 1982; 17:1259–1271.

17. Mills EJ, Noyes HL. Pattern and correlates of initial and subsequent drug use among adolescents. J Consul Clin Psychol. 1984; 52:231–243.

18. Udell JC, Smith RS, Edwards CS. Attitudes and the usage of other drugs and nonusers of marijuana in a high school population. *Wisconsin Project Report,* Vol. 4, 1969.

19. Bauman KE. *Predicting Adolescent Drug use: Utility structure and marijuana.* New York: Praeger Publishers, 1980.

20. Kandel DB, Kessler RC, Margulies RZ. Antecedents of adolescent initiation into stages of drug use: A developmental analysis. In D. B. Kandel (Ed.), *Longitudinal research on drug use: Empirical findings and methodological issues.* New York: John Wiley & Sons, 1978.

21. DeRois MD, Feldman DJ. Southern California Mexican American drinking patterns: Some preliminary observations. J Psychedelic Drugs. 1977; 2:151–158.

22. Maddox JF. Characteristics of Mexican American addicts. *Proceedings of the Institute on Narcotic Addiction Among Mexican Americans in the Southwest,* National Institute of Mental Health, April, 1971:21–23.

23. Padilla ER, Padilla AM, Morales A, Olmedo EL, Ramirez R. Inhalant, marijuana and alcohol abuse among Barrio Children and Adolescents Int J Addict. 1979; 14:943–964.

24. Perez R, Padilla AM, Ramirez A, Ramirez R, Rodrigues M. Correlates and changes over time in drug and alcohol use within a Barrio population. *Spanish Speaking Mental Health Research Center,* Occasional Paper No. 9, 1979.

25. Huba GJ, Wingard JA, Bentler PM. Beginning adolescent drug use and peer and adult interaction patterns. J Consul Clin Psychol. 1979; 47:256–276.

26. Lawley DN, Maxwell AE. *Factor analysis as a statistical method.* 2nd Ed. New York: American Elsevier, 1982.

27. Huba GJ, Wingard JA, Bentler PM. A comparison of two latent variable causal models for adolescent drug use, J Pers Soc Psychol. 1981; 40:180–193.

28. Kirk RE. *Experimental design: Procedures for the behavioral sciences.* Belmont, California: Brooks/Cole Publishing Company, 1982.

29. Winer BJ. *Statistical principles in experimental design.* New York: McGraw-Hill Book Company, Inc. 1982.

30. Chitwood DD, Wells KS, Russe BR. Medical and treatment definitions of drug use: The case of adolescent user. Adolesc. 1981; 16(64):817–830

31. Kleinman PH, Lukoff IF. Ethnic differences in factors related to drug use, J Health Soc Behav. 1978; 19:190–199.

32. Medina AS, Wallace HM, Ralph NR, Goldstein H. Adolescent health in Alameda county, J Adoles Health Care 1982; 2:175–182.

33. Newcomb MD, Huba GJ, Bentler PM. Mother's influence on the drug use of their children: Confirmatory tests of direct modeling and mediational theories. Dev Psychol. 1983; 19(5):714–726.

Factors Associated With the Initiation of "Smoking" in Nine Year Old Children

Tian P.S. Oei, PhD
Annette M. Egan, MA
Phil A. Silva, PhD

ABSTRACT. The present study examined the relationship between 787 (415 boys and 372 girls) nine year old children's reported experience with cigarettes and the parents, home environment, peers, socioeconomic status, school performance and behavior or emotional problems and delinquency factors which had in the past been found to be influential during the formative stages of initiation into the use of tobacco. The 787 children (415 boys and 372 girls) were classified as either "puffers" (those who had puffed on a cigarette) or nonpuffers. The results suggest than, at age nine, puffers were more likely than nonpuffers to: (1) intend to smoke in the future; (2) have one or both parents smoking; (3) have one, or more, smoking friend(s); (4) do less well at maths and school work in general; (5) misbehave more often; and (6) be taken to see a psychologist regarding a behavioral or emotional problem.

To date, almost all attempts to scientifically investigate patterns of use of cigarettes among school children and signifi-

Drs. Oei and Silva are with the Dunedin Multidisciplinary Health and Development Research Unit, Department of Pediatrics and Child Health, University of Otago Medical School, Dunedin, New Zealand. Dr. Oei is also affiliated with the Department of Psychology at University of Otago, as is Ms. Egan.

The Dunedin Multidisciplinary Research and Development Unit is supported by the Medical Research Council of New Zealand, the National Children's Health Research Foundation, The McKenzie Education Foundation, and the Departments of Education and Health. It also draws upon the involvement of several departments of the University of Otago. Much of the data is gathered by voluntary workers from the Dunedin community. The authors are indebted to the many people whose contributions make this ongoing study possible.

Requests for reprints to Dr. Oei who is now at the Psychology Clinic, Department of Psychology, Queensland University, St. Lucia, Qld. 4067 Australia.

cant influencing factors have concentrated either on those who have reached the high school level or, rarely, those in the younger age bracket of 10 to 12 years. While some relevant and useful insights have been gained through such projects, there is evidence that for a large proportion of children, initiation into the use of tobacco occurs at a much younger age.[1-5] Recently Oei et al.[6] reported the prevalence of smoking among nine year old children and their attitudes and knowledge of the effects of cigarette smoking on health. While there is no lack of literature from previous studies linking older age (between 10 and 16) children's cigarette consumption and significant environmental and psychosocial factors, there are no studies investigating influencing factors at age nine.

Since the list of factors which could have been included in the present study was potentially very large, only a few considered to be important were examined here. All of those measures examined had previously been shown to be important with teenagers. These were: family attitudes and habits,[4,7,10] home environment, peer influence, socioeconomic status,[1,5,7] school performance[1] and behavioral or emotional problems and delinquency.[11] The main aim of the present project was to examine a number of factors which could be influential during initiation into the use of tobacco by nine year old children.

METHOD

Sample

The data for this report were collected as part of a longitudinal health and developmental research by the Dunedin Multidisciplinary Child Development research unit.[12] The subjects used in this study and their characteristics were similar to those described in our earlier report,[6] and therefore full description of the sample was not expected here. Briefly, the sub-sample represented in this study consisted of 415 boys and 372 girls. These children were interviewed within one month of their ninth birthday.

Assessment Procedure

Prior to interviewing the children about experiences and attitudes towards cigarettes, written consent for such an interview was obtained from the parent who accompanied the child to the study. Children were assured of the confidential nature of the interview and responses were recorded. All interviews were done in a quiet and private area by an interviewer with no parents or observers present. They were carefully structured in the same manner for each child so as to provide as uniform an interview as possible. Assessment sessions went on for a whole morning and part of the afternoon. A maximum of six children were assessed daily. All children were interviewed or assessed on the following scale: (1) the children's questionnaire about smoking,[6] (2) the Discipline Questionnaire[12] which related to general disciplinary measures used by parents in the home, (3) the Rutter Behavior Questionnaire,[13] (4) the Moos Family Environment Scale,[14] (5) the General Health and Medical Questionnaire[12] and (6) the Student's Perception of Abilities Scale.[15]

It should be emphasised that this research project was based solely on the self reports of the sampled children and an accompanying parent. Some of those responding to questions may have been less than accurate and this could have distorted findings to some extent. However since the confidential nature of results was clearly expressed, it was assumed that most of the responses were, in fact, accurate.

RESULTS

Following an earlier report,[6] we decided to divide the children into "puffer" and "nonpuffer" groups. The reasons for such division were explained earlier. The formal definition for the term "puffer" was: "Any child who had, at some time, puffed on a cigarette." A Chi Square analysis was used to determine the relationship of a puffer and the factors investigated.

It should be noted that not all totals displayed in Table 1 include all 787 sampled children. This is because, in many cases, only "Yes" and "No" responses were considered i.e., those who did not reply or answered with "Don't know" were

TABLE 1

Summary of the Relationship Between Children's Puffing
and the Variables Tested and Chi Square Values

Measures	Group		x^2(1 df)
	Puffers N	Non-puffers N	
1. Parents' reported smoking			
Mothers	109 (41.6%)	163 (33.7%)	4.27*
Fathers	115 (47.7%)	162 (37.1%)	6.37*
2. Child's report of parents' smoking			
Mothers	123 (45.1%)	177 (36.0%)	5.70*
Fathers	135 (52.7%)	208 (43.5%)	5.37
3. Peer Influence			
One or more smoking friends	67 (24.6%)	72 (14.5%)	11.37**
4. Number of parents and children's tendency to puff			
Two parent families	236 (86.0%)	454 (93.8%)	5.82*
5. School performance			
Maths performance	201 (73.6%)	321 (65.2%)	7.18**
General school performance	207 (76.4%)	328 (66.7%)	7.90**
6. Frequency of misbehaviour			
One or less	132 (48.5%)	282 (57.6%)	5.42*
7. Referral to psychologist			
Yes	12 (43.9%)	7 (11.7%)	5.31*
8. Sipped alcohol			
Yes	439 (98.7%)	269 (88.5%)	22.75**

$* = p < .01$
$** = p < .001$
df = 1

excluded. A summary of results showing the relationship between puffers and the variables tested is shown in Table 1.

Factors Related to Onset of Smoking

Parental Influence

Both parents and children reported on parental use of cigarettes. The distributions of the two sets of responses showed that in all, 64 percent of mothers and 59 percent of fathers were non-smokers according to parental reports while children claimed that 61 percent of mothers and 54 percent of fathers were non-smokers. Chi Square statistics were calculated in order to test the strength of the relationship between the tendency for children to have puffed on a cigarette and parental patterns of use reported by parents and children.

The results revealed that there was a significant association between child smoking and reports of parental smoking (see Table 1). It appeared that those children from homes where either mother or father used cigarettes, were more likely to have puffed on a cigarette themselves.

Peers

The smoking habits of peers were investigated by asking children "Do any of your friends smoke?" The distribution of their responses showed that most children (81 percent) had no smoking friends. Of the remaining children, almost all (15 percent) had only one friend who smoked, 2 percent had two friends who smoked and 2 percent each had three or four who smoked.

Chi Square analysis was carried out in an attempt to investigate the relationship between peers smoking habits and children's own puffing experience. When all eight peer categories were included (i.e., from no smoking friends to seven smoking friends) the χ^2 value of 1973 was significant (p < .01). When peers were categorised either as puffers or nonpuffers, the results of Chi Square analysis were also significant ($\chi^2 = 11.37$, 1 df, p < .01) indicating that those children who claimed to have smoking friends were much more likely to have tried smoking themselves than those with no smoking friends.

Socioeconomic Status

As previously stated, the present sample was slightly socio-economically advantaged (Oei et al., 1984). Chi Square analysis comparing puffers and nonpuffers across all socioeconomic levels revealed that no significant relationship existed between the tendency for children to have tried cigarettes and their fathers' occupational status.

Performance at School

Two measures of performance at school were considered. These were, firstly, level of school performance as reported by parents, and, secondly, the child's own perceived level of performance in comparison with the others in his/her class. Most parents (61.6 percent) seemed to believe that their children's level of achievement at school was generally fairly average, with 37.6 percent saying their child was above average and 7.6 percent classifying their child as slow.

A total of 40 percent of the children answered "Yes" to the item "I am one of the brightest kids in the class" compared with 60 percent who believed they were not one of the brightest. Chi Square tests were used to analyse the strength of the relationship between the tendency for children to have puffed on a cigarette and their parents' reports of their school achievement. While reading, printing and writing, and spelling performance were not related to the child's smoking, there was a significant association between puffing and how well the child was seen to be getting on with mathematics ($\chi^2 = 7.2$, 1 df, p $< .01$). Similarly, general school performance and puffing were also closely related ($\chi^2 = 7.9$, 1 df, p $< .01$).

Thus it appeared that nonpuffers were perceived as doing better on mathematics in particular and school work in general, than puffers according to parental reports of school performance. However, children's own perceptions of how well they did in class were not significantly associated with puffing.

Behavioral and Emotional Problems and Delinquency

Four measures were taken as indicators of behavioral and emotional problems. Firstly, parents were asked to indicate how many times yesterday their child was/did: rude/obstinate or disobedient/destructive/silly or showed off/agressive/demanding or whining or nagging/untidy/steal something/told a lie/broke a promise/did anything dangerous/made a nuisance by being overactive. Responses were totalled and just over half of the parents (54 percent) claimed that their children had either been no problem on the previous day or had only misbehaved once, 68 percent of the children had misbehaved twice or less, and 79 percent three times or less. When those who had been a problem only once or not at all were compared with the rest, a Chi Square test revealed an association with puffing experience ($\chi^2 = 5.4$, 1 df, p < .01). Nonpuffers misbehaved significantly less than puffers.

The second measure investigated the difficulty parents had in managing their child. Altogether, 8.0 percent of parents had children who were described as being "difficult to manage." No significant relationship was found between being "difficult to manage" and children's puffing using Chi Square tests. This was also the case with the third measure which involved asking parents to indicate the frequency of children's temper tantrums. For 91 percent this was less than once a month.

Finally, parents were required to think back over the past four years since their child had started school. They were then asked to indicate whether, in that period, they had sought help or advice for a behavior or emotional problem from any one of a number of health or social agencies including general practitioners, Social Welfare, and so on.

When visits to the various agencies were considered overall, there were no differences between puffers and nonpuffers. In most of the subcategories, e.g., visits to health nurse, numbers were too small for meaningful comparisons. The one significant finding was that those children who had been taken to see an educational psychologist because of a behavioral or emotional problem were much more likely to have tried a puff of a cigarette than those who had not ($\chi^2 = 5.3$, 1 df, p < .01).

In summary, puffers were more likely than nonpuffers to have misbehaved more than once on the day prior to assessment and to have been taken to an educational psychologist within the last four years regarding a behavioral or emotional problem.

Family Environment

Two measures of family environment were taken and analysed in order to ascertain whether a relationship existed between this environment and puffing of cigarettes in children. The first of these measures was the "Moos Family Environment Scale" which was divided into 10 individual subscales. There were no significant relationships between children's puffing and any of the Moos subscales so these results are not reported in detail.

The number of parents and parental figures each child has had and the stability of the family (i.e., "how many changes in parent figures has child had?") were taken together as the second measure of the home environment. Altogether 11 percent of children lived in homes with only one parent and 17 percent had not always had the same two parent figures. Chi Square values showed that nonpuffers were much more likely to come from two parent families than were puffers ($\chi^2 = 5.8$, 1 df, p < .01).

In summary, when both measures of family environment were considered together, nonpuffers were more likely to come from two parent homes than puffers.

Puffing Experience and Alcohol Experience

The cross tabulation of puffers and sippers of alcohol is presented in Table 1. A chi-square value was calculated and the results showed that those children who had tried puffing were most likely to be those who had also tasted alcohol and vice versa ($\chi^2 = 22.35$, 1 df, p < .01).

DISCUSSION

Results from previous studies of children aged from 10 to 18 years have indicated that parents' and children's smoking habits are closely related.[4, 7, 9] When the relationship between the tendency for children in the present sample to have puffed on a cigarette and parental patterns of use was examined, findings supported those of other researchers. Puffers were more likely to have at least one smoking parent than nonpuffers.

According to Babst et al.,[16] Tudor,[10] Adler and Lotecka[17] there is a strong and significant association between the type of home environment a child lives in and his/her tendency to have tried many types of drugs. The findings of this study revealed that there was no significant relationship between puffers and nonpuffers and the type of home environment in which a child lives.

Closely related to the type of home environment was the question of what effects single parent families had on children's tendency to have tried smoking. While none of the environmental measures just mentioned were related to puffing cigarettes in this study, nonpuffers were much more likely to come from two parent homes than puffers. Such a distinction had previously been found between regular smoking and non smoking children.[5]

It is suggested that friends often play a critical role in encouraging a child to try the first cigarette. This was supported by the results of this study, which indicated that there was a strong tendency for puffers to have more smoking friends than nonpuffers. However, overall, the number of those children who did have smoking peers (19.2 percent) was much less than those reported by Rawbone et al.[9] and Lemin,[4] whose investigations had dealt with older children.

Evidence presented in this study did not support the findings of O'Connell et al.,[5] Salber and MacMahon[7] who showed that children whose fathers were manual workers or came from lower socio-economic groups were more likely to smoke and/or drink alcohol than those who had fathers working in non-manual occupations or fathers from higher socio-economic groups. For the children sampled here, there were no significant differences between the socioeconomic levels of puffers and nonpuffers.

School achievement scores and smoking in children are related, according to Salber, MacMahon and Welsh[7] and many others. This was the case for the children in this study. When parents reported on performance at school, results showed that nonpuffers did better on maths in particular and school work in general than puffers.

When puffers and nonpuffers were considered, puffers were more likely to have misbehaved on the day prior to assessment. They had also more frequently been taken to see an educational psychologist within the last four years regarding a behavioral or emotional problem. This evidence supported that produced by Lettieri and Ludford[11] who claimed that some predictive factors of early drug involvement are behavior disorders, aggressiveness, and rebelliousness.

Thus, in conclusion, it appeared that many of the factors investigated were significantly associated with children's experience with cigarettes and alcohol. The extent to which the influence they exerted was independent of other variables was not examined and may provide an interesting starting point for future research.

SUMMARY

From the present results, it was possible to draw a general profile of the puffer in the present sample as compared with the nonpuffer.

Puffers were significantly more likely to:

1. have one or both parents smoking
2. have one or more smoking friends
3. do less well at maths and school work in general
4. come from single parent homes
5. misbehave more often, and
6. be taken to see a psychologist regarding a behavior or emotional problem.

REFERENCES

1. Bewley BR, Beulah R, Bland JM. Academic performance and social factors related to cigarette smoking by school children. *Brit. J. Preventative and Social Medicine*, 1977; 31: 18–24.

2. Levitt EE, Edwards JA. A multivariate study of correlative factors in youthful cigarette smoking. *Developmental Psychology*, 1970; 2: 5-11.

3. Levine EM, Kozak C. Drug and alcohol use, delinquency, and vandalism among upper middle class pre- and post-adolescents. *J. Youth and Adolescence*, 1979; 8: 91–101.

4. Lemin B. Smoking in 14-year-old children. *Int. J. of Nursing Studies*, 1967; 4: 301–307.

5. O'Connell PL, Alexander HM, Dobson AJ, Lloyd DM, Hardes GR, Springthorpe HJ, Leeder SR. Cigarette smoking and drug use in school children. Eleven factors associated with smoking. *Int. J. of Epidemiology*, 1981; 10: 223–231.

6. Oei TPS, Brasch P, Silva PA. The prevalance of "smoking" among Dunedin nine year olds and their knowledge of the health and other implications of cigarette smoking. *NZ Medical Journal* 1984; 97: 528–531.

7. Salber, EJ, Macmahon B, Welsh B. Smoking habits of high school students related to intelligence and achievement. *Pediatrics*, 1962; 29: 780–787.

8. Rawbone RG, Keeling CA, Jenkins A, Guz A. Cigarette smoking among secondary school children in 1975. *J. Epidemiology and Community Health*, 1978; 32: 53–58.

9. Rawbone RG, Keeling CA, Jenkins A, Guz A. Cigarette smoking among secondary school children in 1975: its prevalence and some of the factors that promote smoking. *Health Education Journal*, 1979; 38: 92–99.

10 Tudor CG, Petersen CM, Elifson KW. An examination of the relationship between peer and parental influences and adolescent drug use. *Adolescence*, 1980; 15: 783–798.

11. Lettieri DJ, Ludford JP. Drug abuse and the American adolescent. *National Institute on Drug Abuse Research Monograph Series*, 1981; 38.

12. McGee R, Silva PA. A Thousand New Zealand Children: Their health and development from birth to seven. *Medical Research Council of NZ*. Special Report Series No. 8. 1982.

13. Rutter M, Tizard J, Whitmore K. *Education, Health and Behavior*, London, Longman, 1970.

14. Moos, R. Combined Preliminary Manual for the Family: Work and Group Environment Scale. Palo Alto, Consulting Psychologists Press, 1974

15. Boersma FJ, Chapman JA. *Students's Perception of Ability*, Edmonton, University ot Alberta, 1979.

16. Babst DV, Sherry D, Schmeidler J, Dembo R. A study of family affinity and substance use. *J. of Drug Education*, 1978; 8: 29–40.

17. Adler D, Lotecka L. Drug use among high school students: Patterns and correlates. *Int. J. of Addictions*, 1973; 8: 537–548.

Onset of Adolescent Drinking: A Longitudinal Study of Intrapersonal and Interpersonal Antecedents

Judith S. Brook, EdD
Martin Whiteman, PhD
Ann Scovell Gordon, MA
Carolyn Nomura, MA
David W. Brook, MD

ABSTRACT. This study investigated several models for exploring the interrelationships of domains of personality, peer, and family factors and their effect on initiation into alcohol use. Three hundred eighteen black and white high school students were administered questionnaires when they were in the ninth and tenth grades (T1) and again two years later when the students were in the eleventh and twelfth grades (T2). Only those students who had never used alcohol at T1 were included in this study. The results supported an independent model: Each of the domains of T1 personality, peer, and family factors, with control on the other domains, had a direct effect on T2 initiation into alcohol use. The interactions of peer variables with personality and family variables were examined. The findings indicated that risk factors stemming from the peer group were ameliorated by protective personality and family factors.

Judith S. Brook, Ann Scovell Gordon, Carolyn Nomura, and David W. Brook are with the Department of Psychiatry, Mount Sinai School of Medicine, New York, NY. Martin Whiteman is at the School of Social Work, Columbia University, New York, NY.

This study was supported by Public Health Service Grant DA01097-07 (Scope C) (Irving Lukoff, Principal Investigator: Judith Brook, Co-Principal Investigator) from the National Institute on Drug Abuse to the Center for Socio-Cultural Research on Drug Use, Columbia University.

The authors thank Dr. Dan Lettieri for his encouragement and support. They are also grateful for the contributions of the late June Esserman, who was responsible for data collection, and for the essential research assistance of Sandy Stillman.

Requests for reprints should be sent to Judith S. Brook, Mt. Sinai School of Medicine, 1 Gustave Levy Place, Annenberg 22-74, New York, New York 10029.

INTRODUCTION

In past research on the use of alcohol by adolescents, considerable attention has been devoted to the impact of intrapersonal (personality) and interpersonal (family and peer) influences. Evidence obtained in several studies on intrapersonal factors indicates that alcohol use during adolescence is associated with attitudes of nonconformity or nonconventionality and deviant behavior.[1-5] Adolescent alcohol use has also been found to be inversely related to academic achievement and motivation.[1-3,6] Within the family area, greater parental alcohol use[3-7] and certain kinds of parent-adolescent relations (e.g., less affectionate, more rejecting[8]) have been found to be associated with the adolescent's use of alcohol. Past studies have not focused on the effect of sibling alcohol use, although the impact of the sibling on the adolescent's use of other drugs has received increased attention in recent years (e.g., Brook, Whiteman, Gordon, and Brenden[9]). Within the peer area, peer alcohol use, peer approval of drinking, and the youngster's closeness to the peer group have been found to have an impact on his/her use of alcohol.[1-7]

Both theory and research suggest that there are three crucial psychosocial processes that underlie interpersonal influences—modeling, identification, and social reinforcement. Modeling refers to the direct imitation of another's behavior. Although identification has been defined in various ways, Bandura[10] contends that ". . . it is generally agreed that identification refers to a process in which a person patterns his thoughts, feelings or actions after another person who serves as a model" (p. 214). Identification differs from simple modeling in that it involves the conscious or unconscious motive to be like another rather than the direct imitation of the other's specific behaviors. Social reinforcement is the process whereby a person receives positive and negative social reinforcement for specific behaviors. Social reinforcement may directly affect the adolescent's behavior without changing certain aspects of personality, such as some underlying motives or values. Social reinforcement would of course minimize the theoretical importance of the adolescent's own personality attributes. On the other hand, successful socialization may require adolescent personality processes that involve a gradual substitution of symbolic and internal control for external sanctions and demands.

Several investigators have highlighted the importance of examining interrelations among significant aspects of the adolescent's life simultaneously, in order to obtain as complete a picture as possible of adolescent development and behavior, and to determine the relative impact of these different aspects (e.g., Brook, Lukoff, and Whiteman,[11] Jessor and Jessor,[2] Kandel[3]). To accomplish this in the present study, an approach previously used in the examination of adolescent marijuana use will be employed.[11] This approach involves the examination of three alternative models (independent, interdependent, and mediational), in order to see which one best describes the interrelationship of three domains (personality, family, and peer) and their effect on adolescent initiation into alcohol use.

In the case of the *independent* model, all three domains would be significantly related to initiation into alcohol use with and without control on one another, indicating that the personality, family, and peer domains each have an independent impact on initiation into adolescent alcohol use. If all three domains were significant without control, but each lost significance with control on the other domains, this would support an *interdependent* model, suggesting that variables from all three domains coexist in their significant impact on alcohol use. Lastly, if the three domains were significant without control, but only one remained significant with control on the other two domains, this would support a *mediational* model, in which one domain is *prepotent* to the others and mediates their relationship to alcohol use. For example, if the personality domain remained significant but the family and peer domains did not, this would suggest that family and peer attributes affect the child's personality, which in turn affects his/her initiation into alcohol.

Another purpose of this study is to examine the interactions among specific variables as contrasted with the broader domain analysis cited above. Since peer group factors have been found to have a considerable effect on later initiation into the use of alcohol, the extent to which these peer group influences can be ameliorated by other aspects of the adolescent's life was considered to be of interest. Therefore, we examined whether specific personality and family *protective* factors could offset the effects of specific peer *risk* factors in terms of the adolescent's alcohol initiation. What we are designating as personality and family protective factors are those variables that have been found in past research (our own, as well as others') to be related to less adolescent legal or illegal drug use, as either main or interactive effects. These would include personality variables such as conventionality and achievement, and family variables such as good parent-child relations and parental nonuse of drugs. Peer risk factors are those found in the past to be related to more adolescent drug use and include such variables as peer drug use and peer deviance. (It should be noted that protective and risk designations represent opposite ends of the same continuum. For example, conventionality and good parent-child relations are protective characteristics, whereas unconventionality and poor parent-child relations are risk factors.) In sum, we will examine the combined impact on adolescent alcohol initiation of individual peer risk variables with personality and family protective variables. Based on previous research, our hypothesis is that risk factors in the adolescent's peer environment can be ameliorated (offset) by protective factors in his/her own personality or family environment resulting in less likelihood of alcohol initiation.

Finally, this study investigates the differences among nonusers, initiates who are experimental drinkers, and initiates who are regular users, in terms of their prior personality traits and interpersonal influences. Personality variables such as depression and rebelliousness have been identified by Jones[12,13] as differentiating among abstainers, moderate, and problem drinkers. Parent and peer influences have also been found to be associated with frequency of alcohol use.[7]

In sum, the purpose of the present study is to explore the following: first, how do domains of personality attributes, family influences, and peer influences interrelate in terms of the adolescent's initiation into the use of alcohol; second, how do specific protective factors, drawn from the family and personality domains, offset alcohol risk conditions stemming from the peer group, and third, what are the causal factors involved in differential levels of alcohol consumption among nonusers, experimental users, and regular users in adolescence?

A major advantage of the present study is the use of a

prospective longitudinal design in which intrapersonal attributes and interpersonal influences were obtained before the subjects' initiation into alcohol use. This enables us to assert with greater confidence that these effects determined alcohol use rather than resulted from it.

METHODS

Subjects

The original sample at T1 consisted of 403 black and 529 white students with approximately equal numbers of males and females. The subjects were all high school freshmen or sophomores and attended predominantly middle class urban public schools located in Connecticut, Kansas, New Jersey, New York, Ohio, and South Carolina. The schools were carefully selected to ensure a socioeconomically matched sample of black and white students. Two years later (T2), the students were seen again when they were juniors/seniors, at which time 706 (76% of the original sample) youngsters participated again. Sample attrition was due mainly to inability to locate subjects. Only about 5% refused to participate again at T2. The results of a series of T tests on the independent variables in this study revealed that drop-outs (those who participated only at T1) differed from continuing subjects on a number of T1 personality, peer, and family measures. The findings indicated that continuing subjects in comparison to drop-outs were more conventional, more achievement-oriented, less involved in drugs and deviance, were from "intact" homes, and involved in conventional and non-drug-using peer groups. A more detailed presentation of this analysis appears elsewhere.[14]

Of the 706 students at T2, only those who had reported at T1 that they had never used alcohol (beer, wine, hard liquor) were included in the present study of alcohol initiation. This reduced the sample to 318 (91 black males, 96 black females, 63 white males, 68 white females).

Procedure

At both points in time, students were asked to volunteer for the study through letters to parents and students distrib-

uted through the schools. Parental as well as student signed
informed consent forms were required for participation in the
study. A fee of $5.00 was paid to the student at each time for
his/her participation. Some students were paid directly; however, some schools requested that the money be donated to
school funds.

Data collection was similar at both points in time and was
done mostly by Hyatt Esserman Research Associates. The
students were administered written questionnaires in small
group sessions. The questionnaires contained closed-ended
items and took about one hour to complete. Since this was a
longitudinal study, the students were asked to put their names
on face sheets attached to the questionnaires. The face sheets
were removed immediately after they were handed in; only
code numbers were on the questionnaires themselves. A
"Certificate of Confidentiality" was issued by the United
States Department of Justice providing legal protection regarding confidentiality. The subjects were informed accord-
ingly, so they could be sure their responses to the questionnaires would be anonymous.

Measures

The T1 and T2 questionnaires were virtually identical and
contained items designed to assess personality, family, and
peer variables. The family and peer measures were based on
the youngster's perceptions of these aspects of his/her life—no
actual data were obtained from family and peers. The questionnaire items were eventually grouped into scales based on
their intercorrelations and reliabilities. Factor analysis was
also used to reduce the data set and to increase scale reliabilities. For the most part, the scales were adaptations of existing
scales with adequate psychometric properties. The measures
and their sources are listed below.* The scale reliabilities reported are for T1 since these are the measures used in this
paper. The scale reliabilities at T2 were quite similar.

Domain of Adolescent Personality Measures. The scales included in this domain were Tolerance of Deviance/ Risk-Tak-

---

*For a more complete description of the measures, see Brook, Whiteman, and
Gordon.[15]

ing,[16,17] Achievement Orientation,* Orientation to Work,[16] Rebelliousness,[18] Depression,[19]and Self-Deviance.[20] Reliabilities (Cronbach alphas) ranged from .65 to .82 with a median of .76.

Domain of Family Measures. The scales used for this domain were Paternal Warmth, Paternal Permissiveness, Father's Expectations for Child, Maternal Warmth, Maternal Negative-Rejecting Behavior, Maternal Permissiveness,[21,22] Maternal and Paternal Identification, Parental Harmony, Family Expectations.[17] and Parent vs. Peer. Reliabilties ranged from .56 to .93 with a median of .72. Also included in the family domain were measures of parental use of cigarettes, alcohol, and marijuana, and prescribed use of amphetamines, barbiturates, and tranquilizers. In addition, a measure of sibling drug use was included.

Domain of Peer Measures. The scales in this domain included Warmth and Negative-Rejecting Behavior,[21] Deviance,[20] Time Spent with Friends, Identification with Peers, and Number of Achievement-Oriented Friends. Reliabilities ranged from .56 to .91 with a median of .72. Also included in the peer domain were measures of peer marijuana use, peer legal drug and peer illegal drug use (other than marijuana, which was measured separately).

The dependent variable, alcohol initiation, was based on the subject's responses to two questions asked at T2. The first question was "During the past two years, how often did you drink beer or wine?" The second question was identical but asked about "alcohol, that is, hard liquor." The two-year time period was, of course, based on the amount of time that had elapsed between the two waves of the study. There were five response options for both questions: (1) never; (2) 3 times a month or less; (3) once a week to several times a week; (4) 1 or 2 drinks every day; and (5) 3 or more drinks every day. The responses to the two items were summed so that the scores ranged from 2 (nondrinkers at T2) to 10 (3 or more drinks every day for beer/wine and hard liquor). As stated earlier, all subjects were nondrinkers at T1. At T2 the usage rates for initiation into alcohol use were low (mean use

---

*The Achievement Orientation scale was developed by the authors, as were the Maternal and Paternal Identification, Parental Harmony, Parent vs. Peer, Time Spent with Friends, Identification with Peers, and Number of Achievement-Oriented Friends scales. Copies of these scales are available on request.

= 2.95, *SD* = 1.08). This group as a whole can be described as just beginning experimentation with alcohol.

RESULTS

Before carrying out the major analyses, we needed to determine whether there were any significant demographic (i.e., sex, race, socioeconomic status) interactive effects. Regressions were run in which the interactions of each T1 personality, family and peer measure with each demographic variable were examined. The dependent variable was intiation to alcohol use. Only two interactions out of 105 were significant, so the remaining analyses were done on the entire sample.

Correlates of Initiation

Pearson correlations were computed between the T1 adolescent personality, family, and peer variables and T2 initiation into adolescent alcohol use. The results are presented in Table 1. As shown in Table 1, while all of the personality attributes predicted initiation, the highest correlations were obtained for less orientation to work, tolerance of deviance, and deviance. With respect to the family variables, initiates in comparison to noninitiates were more likely to report greater parental permissiveness and less maternal identification. They were also more likely to report greater sibling drug use, paternal drinking, and maternal use of amphetamines, barbiturates, or tranquilizers. As to the peer correlates of alcohol initiation, the highest correlations were obtained for peer drug use, both legal and illegal, and peer deviance.

Domain Interrelationships

In order to see which of the three hypothesized models (independent, interdependent, mediational) best described the data, hierarchical multiple regression analysis was used to examine the interrelations of domains of personality, family, and peer variables, and their impact on initiation into alcohol use. This technique enables one to examine the effect of a specific domain (set of variables) with control by partialing out the effects of the other sets.[23] For example, in examining the impact of personality factors, in one regression the personality domain was entered first (without control). In another regression the family and peer domains were entered into the regression first (as controls) followed by the set of personality variables. A similar procedure was used to examine the effects of the peer and family variables. The results of the analyses are shown in Table 2. As can be seen in Table 2, each of the three domains was significantly related to initiation both without and with control on the remaining sets. The findings therefore supported an independent model in which each domain of personality, family, and peer factors had a direct effect on the adolescents' initiation into use of alcohol. The three domains of personality, family, and peer factors explained 27 percent of the variance in alcohol initiation.

Combined Effects of Individual Personality Protective and Peer Risk Factors

In order to examine whether personality protective factors could offset peer risk factors in terms of alcohol initiation, two-way analyses of variance were computed. In each ANOVA, the two factors were one personality and one peer variable, each dichotomized into a high and low group. The dependent variable was the continuous measure of initiation to alcohol use. Each personality variable was examined in interaction with each peer variable. Simple effects analyses were done for the significant interactions.* The results are shown in Table 3. As Table 3 shows, protective personality attributes in the adolescent did serve as a buffer against drinking for risk conditions in the adolescent's peer group. For example, high achievement on the part of the adolescent offset the effects of drug use by peers.

Combined Effects of Individual Family Protective and Peer Risk Factors

Two-way analyses of variance followed by simple effects tests were computed as described above for each family variable by each peer variable. A summary of the significant in-

---

*In order to minimize the chance aspects of dealing with a number of significant interactions, first the total number of potential interactions was calculated, e.g., personality × peer (6 personality × 9 peer = 54). Assuming that four types of interaction are possible (personality protective × peer protective; personality protective × peer risk, personality risk × peer protective; personality risk × peer risk), one would expect 13.5 (54/4) interactions of each type to occur. At the .05 level of significance, on would expect 5% (1 out of 13.5) of each type of interaction to be significant Our results showed that 37% (5 out of 13.5) of the personality protective × peer risk interactions were significant.

Table 1

Correlations Between T1 Personality, Family, and Peer
Scales and T2 Initiation to Alcohol Use

Scale	Initiation to alcohol use r
A. Personality Variables	
Tolerance of deviance/risk-taking (more)	.23***
Achievement orientation (less)	.13**
Orientation to hard work (less)	.32***
Rebelliousness/impulsivity (more)	.12*
Depressive mood (more)	.12*
Self-deviance (more)	.19***
B. Family Variables	
Paternal warmth (less)	.03
Paternal permissiveness (more)	.10*
Father's expectations for child (less)	.04
Maternal warmth (more)	.03
Maternal negative-rejecting behavior (more)	.04
Maternal permissiveness (more)	.15**
Parental harmony (more)	.02
Identification with father (less)	.06
Identification with mother (less)	.10*
Family expectations (more)	.03
Sibling drug use (more)	.18***
Maternal drinking	.00
Paternal drinking (more)	.10*

(Table continues on next page)

(Table 1 continued)

Scale	Initiation to alcohol use r
Paternal smoking (less)	.08
Maternal smoking (less)	.06
Paternal marijuana use (less)	.04
Maternal marijuana use	.01
Paternal amphetamine, barbiturate, tranquilizer use	.00
Maternal amphetamine, barbiturate, tranquilizer use (more)	.10*
Parent vs. peer orientation (peer oriented)	.08
C. Peer Variables	
Warmth	.01
Deviance (more)	.11*
Negative-rejecting behavior (more)	.03
Time spent with friends (more)	.07
Identification with friends (more)	.11*
Number of achieving friends (fewer)	.07
Friend legal drug use (more)	.18***
Friend illegal drug use (more)	.10*
Friend marijuana use (more)	.26***

*p < .05

**p < .01

***p < .001

Table 2

Multiple Rs Between T1 Personality, Family, and
Peer Domains and T2 Initiation to Alcohol Use

Domain	R without control		R with control	
	R	F	R	F
A. Personality	.38	8.36**	.32	8.33**
B. Family	.35	2.05**	.25	1.62*
C. Peer	.30	3.41**	.20	2.00*

Note. The variables within the domains are listed in Table 1.

*p < .05

**p < .01

Table 3

Significant Two-Way Interactions (T1 Peer Variables
X Personality Variables X Alcohol Initiation)

| Peer Risk Condition | Adolescent Personality Interactive Effect | | Two-Way Interaction | |
	Lesser initiation Protective Condition	Greater initiation Augmented Risk Condition	F	df
More deviant friends	High achievement	Low achievement	13.08***	1,312
More nonachieving friends	High achievement	Low achievement	4.66*	1,300
More marijuana-using friends	High achievement	Low achievement	5.21*	1,307
More illegal drug-using friends	Low self-deviance	High self-deviance	4.27*	1,292
More marijuana-using friends	Low self-deviance	High self-deviance	7.52**	1,307

Note. Youngsters with peer risk conditions were less likely to initiate alcohol use if their own personalities were "protective" than if they were not. For example, in row one, simple effects tests revealed that in the "deviant friend" condition, the youngster's high achievement was associated with lesser initiation, whereas low achievement was associated with greater initiation.

*$p < .05$ **$p < .01$ ***$p < .001$

teractions appears in Table 4.* As shown in the table, the impact on alcohol initiation of risk conditions in the adolescent's peer group was offset by protective family factors—lack of drug models in the adolescent's family, as well as by a positive parent-child relationship. For instance, low maternal rejection protected the adolescent from the risk effect of having nonachieving friends.

Frequency of Alcohol Use
(Nonuse, Experimental Use, and Regular Use)

A three-group multiple discriminant function analysis was performed to determine the specific T1 family, peer, and personality factors related to different degrees of involvement in T2 consumption of alcohol. The predictor battery contained the independent variables used in the multiple regression analyses (see Table 1). The dependent variable groups were non-users (141), experimental users (less than weekly) = 155, and regular users (once a week or more) = 22. Two functions were significant ($p < .05$), and their canonical correlations were .48 and .29 respectively. The findings indicated that nonusers, experimental users, and regular users of alcohol could be distinguished from one another on a configuration of personality and peer factors. The highest significant standardized discriminant coefficients for the first function included low orientation to work (.64), self-deviance (.51), peer deviance (.44), and peer drug use (.40). Regular users were least work oriented and most deviant, and were the most involved in drug-using peer groups. In contrast, the nonusers were the most work oriented, least deviant, and least involved in drug-using peer groups. The characteristics of the experimental users were in between those of the nonusers and regular users. The highest significant standardized discriminant coefficients for the second function included father warmth (.37) parental harmony (.56), less drug use by siblings (.38), less use of legal drugs by friends (.57) and less paternal alcohol use (.34). Nonusers and experimental users were more likely

---

*Using the calculations described earlier, one would expect 2 of each type of family × peer interaction to occur at the .05 level. Results showed that 27% (12 out of 45) of family protective by peer risk interactions were significant.

Table 4

Significant Two-Way Interactions (T1 Peer Variables
X Family Variables X Alcohol Initiation)

Peer Risk Condition	Family Interactive Effect		Two-Way Interaction	
	Lesser initiation Protective Condition	Greater initiation Augmented Risk Condition	F	df
More nonachieving friends	Low maternal rejection	High maternal rejection	6.85**	1,290
More rejecting friends	Low maternal permissiveness	High maternal permissiveness	4.22*	1,299
More marijuana-using friends	Low maternal permissiveness	High maternal permissiveness	6.55**	1,298
More marijuana-using friends	High father identification	Low father identification	5.64*	1,286
More legal drug-using friends	High mother identification	Low mother identification	4.11*	1,297
More marijuana-using friends	High family expectations	Low family expectations	6.70**	1,305
More deviant friends	Less maternal amphs, etc.¹	More maternal amphs, etc.	12.13***	1,314
Low peer identification	Less maternal amphs, etc.	More maternal amphs, etc.	5.89*	1,313
More nonachieving friends	Less maternal amphs, etc.	More maternal amphs, etc.	9.30**	1,303
More legal drug-using friends	Less maternal amphs, etc.	More maternal amphs, etc.	7.17***	1,309
More marijuana-using friends	Less maternal amphs, etc.	More maternal amphs, etc.	4.85*	1,310
More marijuana-using friends	Parent oriented	Peer oriented	4.43*	1,302

Note. Youngsters with peer risk conditions were less likely to initiate alcohol use if their families were protective than if they were not. For example, in row one, simple effects tests revealed that in the "nonachieving friends" condition, the youngsters who had mothers who were not rejecting were less likely to initiate alcohol use than those whose mothers were rejecting.

¹ amphetamine, barbiturate, or tranquilizer use

*$p < .05$ **$p < .01$ ***$p < .001$

to have an affectionate relationship with their fathers in the context of a harmonious home where models for nonuse of alcohol and drugs were present. In contrast, the regular users of alcohol were more likely to report an unaffectionate relationship with their fathers, parental conflict, and models for the use of alcohol and drugs.

DISCUSSION

Since each of the domains of personality, family, and peer factors had a direct effect on initiation into alcohol use despite control on one another, an independent model best described the interrelationship of the three domains and its impact on the adolescent's alcohol initiation. An implication of this model is that interpersonal factors (family, peer) are not mediated by one another or by the adolescent's intrapersonal qualities, but rather have a direct effect on initiation into alcohol use. Similarly, intrapersonal influences have direct consequences for alcohol initiation without operating through interpersonal influences. Etiologically then, there appear to be different causal pathways leading to the use of alcohol. One therefore cannot say that initiation into alcohol results solely from interpersonal (family, peer) processes on the one hand or from intrapersonal processes on the other. Rather, any one of these processes may be sufficient in and of itself to cause initiation. From the perspective of prevention, as an example, certain family conditions may be helpful in preventing initiation into alcohol; however, deviant peer group influences or personality disturbances may have their own independent effects and lead to initiation. (Further evidence for the independent importance of each of the domains emerged from the discriminant function analysis. Results there indicated that variables from each of the domains loaded on the discriminant functions, e.g., parental conflict from the family domain, low achievement from personality, and peer drug use and deviance from the peer.)

Although we have highlighted the independent impact of each domain, this is not to deny the fact that when negative influences from all the domains are combined, there is increased probability for later alcohol initiation. The proportion of variance contributed when all three domains served as predictors was much greater than the variance contributed by each domain by itself.

Our confidence in the causal impact of these domains on alcohol use is bolstered by the fact that the measures in the intrapersonal and interpersonal domains preceded the use of alcohol and therefore could not have been caused by its use. This is not, of course, to imply that alcohol use does not have an impact on intrapersonal and interpersonal functioning. Previous research does suggest that, at least in the case of compulsive use of alcohol, serious medical, behavioral, and psychosocial consequences can emerge.[24]

The individual personality factors associated with initiation into alcohol use include aspects of nonconventionality or nonconformity. Our results clearly indicated that adolescents who were not work oriented and who did not perform successfully in the academic sphere were indeed more likely to initiate the consumption of alcohol, as were those who were more deviant. These findings are consistent with results of a number of other investigators.[1,2,4,5,25]

The familial environment of the initiates into alcohol use differed from that of the noninitiates in three main ways. First, initiates in comparison to noninitiates reported greater use of drugs by family members, indicating that direct imitation (modeling) of the other's specific behavior is one determinant of the adolescent's own behavior. In line with this, Kandel[26] reported that modeling of parental consumption of distilled spirits was related to both the adolescent's initiation to alcohol and to later phases of alcohol involvement, with the relationship being stronger for the former than for the latter. Alexander and Campbell[7] also found parental drinking to be of importance in their youngster's own drinking. Second, our findings indicated that less (conscious or unconscious) motivation (identification) to be like the mother leads to greater initiation into alcohol use. Previous results in our earlier work showed that maternal nonidentification was positively associated with drug use.[15] Third, our current findings indicated that over-permissiveness on the part of parents is associated with increased alcohol initiation. This appears to corroborate a study by Prendergast and Schaefer,[8] who found that lack of parental control was associated with greater alcohol use by high school seniors.

With regard to the peer influences on alcohol initiation, our findings indicated that peer drug use and deviance were associated with initiation. This is consistent with the findings of several investigators[4-7,26,27] who report that peer modeling (friends' drinking) is an important influence on the adolescent's own drinking behavior.

The present study also highlights the importance of examining the interactions of individual peer risk variables with personality and family protective variables in terms of the adolescent's initiation into alcohol use. As to the interactive effects of personality and peer factors, the findings revealed that the effect of exposure to peer risk factors, such as peer drug use can be ameliorated by protective personality factors in the adolescent. Given friends who were deviant, nonachieving, or involved with marijuana, achievement-oriented and nondeviant youngsters were less likely to initiate alcohol use than were non-achievement-oriented or deviant youngsters.

Combinations of family and peer factors were also shown to have an effect on initiation into alcohol use. As hypothesized, protective family factors offset the influence of exposure to peer risk factors. For example, maternal nonuse of medically prescribed drugs diminished the impact of having friends who were deviant, nonachieving, and who used legal drugs. Another way of looking at this type of interaction would be to emphasize how family risk factors augment peer risk factors. Thus, maternal use of prescribed drugs in conjunction with negative peer group effects increased alcohol initiation. In short, susceptibility to peer risk conditions varied depending on the nature of the familial environment. This supports findings from earlier research on drug use,[28] in which the effects of particular patterns of friends' drug use and deviance were seen to be influenced by the behavior of one's parents. Further, our finding that familial and peer risk factors exacerbated each other is in line with the studies of investigators who have reported that combinations of stressful life events increased the individual's risk of developing physical and mental illness.[29,30]

Overall, our interactive findings suggest that risk conditions in the peer group can be offset by non-drug-prone personality attributes of the adolescent and/or by a non-drug-conducive family environment. An important and heartening implication of these findings is that even if youngsters are exposed to

potent peer risk factors, they will not necessarily become alcohol users.

Finally, it is of interest to note that nonusers, experimental
users, and regular users of alcohol could be differentiated on
a configuration of intrapersonal and interpersonal factors.
The results of the discriminant function analysis suggested
that the three groups differed on a function reflecting adolescent unconventionality and peer engagement in deviance and
drug use. A second function tapping paternal lack of affection
embedded in parental conflict and interpersonal support for
drug use from both family and friends distinguished nonusers
and experimental users from the regular users.

The present study has several limitations. First, the findings
are based on a sample of youngsters who are presently attend-
ing school and may not pertain to adolescents who are not in
school. In addition, as mentioned earlier, the adolescents who
remained in the study at both points in time were systematically different from those youngsters who dropped out of the
study on a number of important variables. For both reasons we
are limited in our ability to generalize to all adolescents. Second, the data relating to interpersonal influences were based
on the adolescent's perceptions of family and peer characteristics. As pointed out by Davies and Kandel,[31] a major
limitation of this approach is that influences may as a consequence be determined in part by the adolescent's own attributes. It is entirely possible that the findings of the present
study would be different if the data on interpersonal influences
had been based on reports obtained from members of the
family and peer group, rather than from the adolescent's perception of these significant others.

Despite these limitations, the results do provide some understanding of the intrapersonal and interpersonal influences
operating on the adolescent's initiation into alcohol use. In
studying domains, the finding of an independent model in
explaining the causal linkages among intrapersonal and interpersonal influences and initiation into alcohol use points to
the direct importance for alcohol use of all these areas of the
youngster's life. In the study of specific variables, we have
shown how particular protective personality traits and family
factors can offset alcohol risk factors stemming from the peer
group.

REFERENCES

1. Jessor R. Collins MI, Jessor SL. On becoming a drinker: Social-psychological aspects of an adolescent transition. Ann NY Acad Sci. 1972; 197:199–213.

2 Jessor R, Jessor, SL. Adolescent development and the onset of drinking: A longitudinal study. J Stud Alcohol. 1975;36:25–51.

3. Kandel DB. Drug and drinking behavior among youth. Annu Rev Sociol. 1980;6:235–286.

4. Kandel D, Kessler R, Margulies R. Adolescent initiation into stages of drug use: A developmental analysis. In: Kandel DB, ed. Longitudinal research on drug use: empirical findings and methodological issues. Washington DC: Hemisphere Publishing Corporation, 1978.

5. Margulies R, Kessler RC, Kandel DB. A longitudinal study of onset of drinking among high school students. Q J Stud Alcohol. 1977;38:897–912.

6. Adler I, Kandel DB. A cross-cultural comparison of sociopsychological factors in alcohol use among adolescents in Israel, France, and the United States. J Youth Adol. 1982;11:89–113.

7. Alexander CN Jr, Campbell EQ. Peer influences on adolescent drinking. Q J Stud Alcohol. 1967;28:444–453.

8. Prendergast TJ Jr, Schaefer, ES Correlates of drinking and drunkenness among high school students. Q J Stud Alcohol. 1974;35:232–242.

9. Brook JS, Whiteman M, Gordon AS, Brenden C. Older brother's influence on younger sibling's drug use. J Psychol. 1983;114:83–90.

10. Bandura A. Social-learning theory of identificatory processes. In: Goslin DA, ed. Handbook of socialization theory and research. Chicago: McNally & Co, 1969:213–262.

11. Brook JS, Lukoff IF, Whiteman M. Initiation into adolescent marijuana use. J Genet Psychol. 1980;137:133–142.

12. Jones MC. Personality correlates and antecedents of drinking patterns in adult males. J Consult Clin Psychol. 1968;32:2–12.

13 Jones MC. Personality antecedents and correlates of drinking patterns in women. J Consult Clin Psychol. 1971;36:61–69.

14. Brook JS, Cohen P, Gordon AS The impact of sample attrition in a longitudinal study of adolescent drug use. Psychol Rep 1983;53:375–378.

15. Brook JS, Whiteman M, Gordon AS. Qualitative and quantitative aspects of adolescent drug use: Interplay of personality, family, and peer correlates Psychol Rep. 1982;51:1151–1163.

16. Jackson DN. Personality research form. Goshen, NY: Research Psychologists Press, 1974.

17. Jessor R, Graves TD, Hanson RC, Jessor SL. Society, personality, and deviant behavior: A study of a tri-ethnic community. New York: Holt, Rinehart, & Winston, 1968.

18. Smith GM, Fogg CP. Psychological antecedents of teenage drug use. In: Simmons R, ed. Research in community and mental health: An annual compilation of research (Vol 1). Greenwich, CT: JAI, 1979;87–102.

19. Derogatis LR, Lipman RS, Rickels K, Uhlenhuth EH, Covi L. The Hopkins Symptom Checklist (HSCL): A self-report symptom inventory. Behav Sci. 1974;19:1–15

20. Gold M. Undetected delinquent behavior. J Res Crime Delinq. 1966;3:27–46.

21. Avgar A, Bronfenbrenner U, Henderson CR Jr. Socialization practices of parents, teachers, and peers in Israel: Kibbutz, moshav, and city. Child Dev. 1977;48.1219–1227.

22. Schaefer ES. Children's report of parental behavior: An inventory. Child Dev. 1965;36:413–424.

23. Cohen J, Cohen P. Applied multiple regression/correlation analysis for the behavioral sciences (2nd ed). Hillsdale NJ: Lawrence Erlbaum Associates, 1983.

24. Diagnostic and statistical manual of mental disorders (DSM III) (3rd ed). Washington DC: American Psychiatric Association, 1982.

25. Wingard JA, Huba GJ, Bentler PM. A longitudinal analysis of personality structure and adolescent substance use. Personality Indiv Diff. 1980;1.259–272.

26. Kandel DB. On processes of peer influences in adolescent drug use: A developmental perspective. Adv Alcohol Substance Abuse. 1985; 4(3/4):139–163.

27. Biddle BJ, Bank BJ, Marlin MM. Parental and peer influence on adolescents. Soc Forces. 1980;58:1057–79.

28. Brook JS, Whiteman M, Gordon AS, Brook DW. Father's influence on his daughter's marijuana use viewed in a mother and peer context. Adv Alcohol Substance Abuse. 1985; 4(3/4):165–190.

29. Dohrenwend BS, Dohrenwend BP, eds. Stressful life events: Their nature and effects. New York: John Wiley, 1974.

30. Rahe RH, Arthur RH. Life change and illness studies: Past history and future directions. J Hum Stress. 1978;4:3–15.

31. Davies M, Kandel DB. Parental and peer influences on adolescents' educational plans: Some further evidence. Am J Sociol. 1981;87:363–387.

Pathways to Heroin Abstinence: A Longitudinal Study of Urban Black Youth

Ann F. Brunswick, PhD
Peter A. Messeri, PhD

ABSTRACT. Reported here is a study of the effectiveness of treatment in reducing the duration of heroin careers, with a special focus on gender differences. The longitudinal research is based on a community representative sample of urban black youth, ages 18–23, and utilizes a recently introduced statistical methodology, event-history analysis. Simple hazard probability analysis confirmed that males and females did not differ significantly in their cumulative probabilities of abstinence from heroin. The more elaborated event-history model demonstrated, however, that treatment played a significantly different role among young men and women in attaining abstinence. While a man's likelihood of abstinence was but marginally greater with treatment than without it, women's likelihood of abstinence was significantly increased by entering treatment.

INTRODUCTION

Empirical research conducted over the last two decades has dispelled the belief that heroin use inevitably results in a permanent state of addiction.[1,2] While precise estimates are lacking, it appears that, for many, heroin addiction is not a lifelong affliction[3-5] and at least some portion of heroin users return to a heroin-free state without benefit of formal treatment.[6-10] The first dramatic evidence that heroin addiction was situation-dependent and spontaneously reversible was provided by Robins[11,12] in her study of drug use among return-

The authors are with Columbia University (Public Health, Sociomedical Services), New York, NY. To request reprints, write: A. Brunswick, PhD, 60 Haven Avenue, B-4, New York, NY 10032.

111

ing Vietnam veterans: the great majority of military personnel who had become addicted in Vietnam discontinued use upon returning to the U.S. The cumulative results of these studies also present strong evidence that heroin users vary considerably in frequency of use and physical dependency. Many individuals have reported using heroin on a casual basis over an extended period of time without (or before) becoming addicted.[3,13,14] Even the heroin careers of addicts are typically interspersed with periods of temporary abstinence.[3,4,15]

If periodic abstinence as well as lasting recovery from heroin abuse are now established phenomena, the same cannot be said for our understanding of the role of treatment in ending heroin careers within a general population of users. Research evaluating the effectiveness of treatment programs has been confined for the most part to the experiences of client populations. Data currently available to distinguish the heroin user most likely to enter treatment[16] and/or to compare patterns of post-treatment abstinence and relapse with the careers of untreated users are indeed limited.

The few studies reviewed by Waldorf and Biernacki[10] which systematically compare treated and untreated heroin users have reported little difference in rates of recovery between the two. Unfortunately, failure to specify clearly the relevant user population along with internal differences between treated and untreated users places severe limits on generalizability from this small body of research. Athough the nonrandom character of treatment entry is well established,[16,17] treated and control groups are rarely matched on salient attributes nor has multivariate analysis been employed to adjust for their differences, differences which when left uncontrolled are likely to confound inferences regarding treatment effects.

Our knowledge is similarly limited when it comes to cross group comparisons of drug treatment efficacy and termination of drug use. The antecedents and functions of heroin use are commonly postulated to differ across broad socioeconomic and demographic categories—ethnicity, sex and age—and by place and time.[2, 18–22] Yet, minimal attention has been paid to systematic comparison of the differential success of treatment in providing for the needs of males *vs.* females; whites *vs.* blacks and/or other minorities; inner-city *vs.* middle-class users. (For an exception, see Savage & Simpson.[23])

In recognition of the dearth of empirical evidence on these matters, this paper selects one particular issue—that of differences in treatment efficacy on the basis of gender. It reports findings from ongoing prospective research into heroin use and treatment behavior in a community sample of nonhispanic black young people (see Methods). The analysis reported here focuses on members of the panel who reported nonexperimental use of heroin for some period of time up to 1976, when the oldest among them still were in their early twenties. The findings can be taken as a representation of heroin experiences of black youths who grew up in Harlem during the 1960s.

In a previous analysis[24] the role of sex and other factors in regulating entry into heroin treatment programs was investigated. Of particular interest, that study demonstrated that female heroin users in the sample tended to enter treatment at a later stage of their careers than males. The present study extends this research to a comparative examination of treatment outcomes: Does treatment intervention reduce the duration of heroin careers relative to the length of careers preceding natural, i.e., untreated abstinence? Retaining emphasis on specifying gender differences in drug related behavior, the question of whether young black male and female heroin users in the study sample differed in their reliance upon treatment as a means of ending their heroin careers is of particular concern. By conducting the analysis within a multivariate framework, simultaneous controls could be imposed on other factors suspected of being associated with either or both treatment entry and the length of heroin careers. Finally, a longitudinal methodology—event-history analysis[25]—has been applied to model the complexities arising from the time varying nature of treatment entry and of certain other conditions hypothesized to influence the duration of heroin use.

STUDY PROBLEM

The present study has been designed to compare annual rates of abstinence achieved through treatment relative to what is achieved without it in a general sample of young black heroin users. Abstinence is defined here as a minimum of one year without use of heroin following a history of nonexperimental use, and without relapse up to the time of second study, i.e., up to ages 18–23. The term "abstinence" was chosen over "cessation" because the latter suggests a more final and permanent state than could be assured at this stage in the longitudinal research. Nor were differences in effects of single and multiple treatment exposures on lengths of abstinence periods at issue in this study, given the relatively young ages and resultant limited variability in number of treatment episodes.

A comparison of treated and untreated abstinence presumes that the length of the heroin careers of untreated users is on average indicative of the duration of use for treated users had they *not entered treatment*. If the assumed comparability of the two populations is valid, then a higher rate of abstinence following treatment would be an indication that treatment did reduce the length of heroin careers below their average "natural" duration. The drug use patterns and practices of treated and untreated users, however, may not be identical. Because of the nonexperimental design of natural fields studies, there is no effective control over self-selection. Systematic differences between treated and untreated users thus may and probably do exist. For example, it is almost certainly true that individuals who enter treatment tend to be more deeply involved in heroin use and find it more difficult to withdraw than natural abstainers.[6] In such a case observed differences in rates of treated and untreated abstinence tend to understate the true effectiveness of treatment.

Other factors, such as the comparatively longer use of heroin and older age of the user entering treatment, are also potential sources of population differences which will confound comparative analysis of rates of treated and natural abstinence. More generally, differential antecedents of the likelihood of abstinence *vs.* treatment entry, if not properly controlled, can bias estimates of treatment effects in an unpredictable direction. Through multiple-regression type analysis, explicit account has been taken in this study of age, frequency of use, and duration of use. These variables were found to affect treatment entry[24] and were considered plausible conditions for influencing the annual probability of abstinence.

A collateral interest in designing this research was to test for gender differences in treatment effects. In the past few years, investigators have begun to take note of gender differences in the psychosocial antecedents and correlates of drug use generally and of heroin use in particular.[20,22,26-30.] Treatment programs, it has been argued frequently, are inattentive to the specific needs of female addicts, particularly in regard to their maternal responsibilities.[18,21,31] Moreover, female addicts may not be as well situated as their male counterparts for terminating use spontaneously, as reflected in their greater impairment of social role performance.[20] If heroin use is a more atypical behavior for black women than men, it may not be unreasonable to suppose that female heroin users are further removed from the intra-individual resources and informal support systems necessary for natural abstinence.

The possible mismatch between the needs of female heroin users and the provisions of treatment services, on the one hand, and their poorer access to natural means of abstinence, on the other, lead to contradictory expectations regarding gender differences in treatment outcome. A greater mismatch in services suggests that treatment would be less efficacious for females than males, whereas poorer access to natural means of abstinence suggests the opposite conclusion. While no attempt was made at this stage of research to confirm either hypothesis directly, the present study takes a first step toward resolving this issue by testing for specific gender differences in treatment outcome. These are reported and discussed below.

METHODS

Source of Data

The data for this study came from the second wave of ongoing research into health and health behavior of an area representative sample of urban, nonhispanic black youth. When originally studied at ages 12–17, the panel was composed of all age appropriate adolescents residing in a cross section of households in Central Harlem (New York City). Households were selected over a two year period (1967–8) through a stratified area probability sample using a four percent (1 in 25) sampling interval each year. The second wave of study was conducted in 1975–6, when the study group were ages 18–23. Ninety-four percent of the original sample of 668 nonhispanic urban black adolescents were located and personal reinterviews were completed with 89 percent of those who were still alive and not found to be residing outside the metropolitan New York City area to which the restudy was limited. This represented 80 percent of the entire initial study group (N = 536). Refusals amounted to but two percent. Males (277) and females (259) were reinterviewed in similar proportions. Approximately two-thirds of the reinterviewed (63%) had remained in Harlem, the others were located primarily in other areas of Manhattan, the Bronx, or Brooklyn.

Interviews both times were conducted in respondents' homes by specially trained, ethnically and gender matched interviewers. Analysis indicates that the reinterviewed sample was well representative of the total initial sample on background and health characteristics.[32]

Extensive drug histories were collected in the second interview as part of a large body of information regarding health status, health practices and living conditions. The drug histories included, for each illicit substance used, age and year of first and last use; frequency of use; recency of use; mode of administration. (See Brunswick[33] for a more complete description of procedures.) In addition, dates of entry and exit into and out of drug treatment programs, environments and modalities of treatment, perceived influences on seeking treatment and other related treatment matters were investigated.[a]

The Sample

Of the total longitudinal panel of 277 males, 18 percent (49) reported experience with heroin and 16 percent (43) reported more than experimental use, i.e., used more than once or twice. Among the 259 females in the panel, 12 percent (30) reported heroin use and ten percent (26) reported more than experimental use. These 43 male and 26 female nonexperimental heroin users comprise the sample for the present study. As should be obvious, this was not a sample of "addicts" but of heroin users who evidenced considerable variability in the patterns of their use. (See first section of Findings below.)

Study Variables

The annual probability of abstaining from heroin use was tested for its association with treatment status, with gender, age, length and frequency of heroin use. The duration of a heroin career was operationally defined as the elapsed time in years between earliest and most recent self-reported use of heroin. No attempt was made to differentiate heroin careers by intermittent spells of abstinence which may have intervened between the two endpoints. Respondents who last used heroin more than a year before reinterview were classified as "abstainers." Those using heroin within a year of reinterview were considered to be current users. Regular frequency of heroin use was coded along a five-point ordinal scale: few times a year/once a month/few times per month/few times per week/every day.

Calendar year of first entry into treatment was the only treatment parameter used in this study. Multiple episodes of treatment, duration of treatment and/or different modalities of treatment were not distinguished, given the small size of the treated sample. For this reason, the test of treatment efficacy reported here probably is conservative and errs in the direction of underestimation, since some experiences classified as treatment were marginal at best—detox, short term, etc. More specifically, 29 percent of the males studied here reported detox as their only treatment experiences.

The specific formulation of the variables for the longitudinal analysis is described below.

Analytical Procedure

The impact of treatment and other conditions hypothesized to influence the duration of heroin careers was examined using event-history analysis. This recent methodological innovation models the relationship between a hazard rate, the annual probability of abstaining, and its covariation with a set of explanatory variables[25,40] (Appendix).

The event history has several features which are advantageous in analyzing longitudinal data:

1. It assumes a dependent variable which reflects a change in discrete state (e.g., from heroin use to abstinence). A dif-

ferent methodology is required when time varying processes assume continuous values.

2. The event-history analysis models a time varying probability, whereby the likelihood of changed state may increase, decrease or remain constant over time. In event-history analysis, these probabilities are expressed as hazard rates. The higher rate corresponds to a greater likelihood of entering the state and thus also denotes an earlier expected entry into the changed state. The independent or model variables measure influences on or proneness to state change by identifying conditions under which state changes are more or less likely to occur.

3. Event-history analysis allows for and can take into account time variations in change in status on explanatory variables against which change in the dependent variable is analyzed. Thus it is particularly appropriate for longitudinal studies. Furthermore, it provides for separation of secular and historic changes (which influence all panel members similarly) from developmental ones (which influence them selectively).

4. Increased power in event-history analysis, relative to more standard regression procedures, derives from retention in study of cases which these other techniques often discard, e.g., those who never enter the changed state. This is the problem of censored data. Increased power also derives from including information on multiple periods of exposure of different individuals. Note that in the present study, once the individual entered the changed state—the most recent year in which s/he used heroin, no later observations were counted, i.e., s/he was no longer considered exposed or at risk.

The unit of analysis for the event-history model was a calendar year. The model was fitted to heroin use experience and data on independent variables observed on an annual basis between 1969 and 1975. The former was the first year any sample member entered treatment and 1975 was the last year an individual could, by definition, have abstained from use for more than a year. An individual was considered at risk of abstaining beginning with first year of use or 1969, whichever came later, through year of last use or 1975.[b]

The independent variables of primary interest were treatment status, gender and an interaction term between treatment status and gender. The treatment status variable was coded "0" for annual observations prior to first-time entry into treatment. The treatment variable was coded "1" in year of first-time entry and all years thereafter. Individuals who never entered treatment were assigned "0" on this variable for all years at risk. Constructed in this way, the treatment status variable measured the difference in the annual hazard probabilities between treated and natural abstinence.

Gender was coded "1" for males and "0" for females. An interaction term between gender and treatment status was included in order to measure the effect of treatment separately for males and females. Alternatively, the interaction term provides separate estimates of gender differences for treated and natural rates of abstinence.

Frequency of heroin use, current age and duration of use were included as control variables. Equal spacing was assumed between the levels of the frequency variables. Age, like treatment status, varied over time and indicated the chronological age at each year of use. This variable controlled for possible increases or declines in the rate of abstinence as users aged. Duration, the length of heroin use, is empirically and conceptually distinct from the probability of abstinence. The variable measured at each annual observation the number of years of use (year of first use was assigned "1") and thus increased by 1 for each year an individual used heroin. Because individuals first used heroin at different ages, the effects of aging and length of use can be simultaneously estimated. The duration variable tests for a systematic increase or decline in the annual probability of abstaining with each additional year of use.

The model was completed by the inclusion of five indicator variables capturing calendar year fluctuations in the probability of abstinence due to unspecified exogenous temporal factors. These coefficients measure deviations from the baseline probability in 1969 for years 1970 through 1975. Since they were included to control for exogenous temporal effects on other variables in the model without inherent substantive meaning, they are not discussed with the findings.

FINDINGS

Patterns of Heroin Use and Treatment Utilization

By ages 18–23 the length of heroin careers varied considerably. Thirty-six percent of males and 26 percent of females reported using heroin for two years or less, while 29 percent of male and 33 percent of female heroin users had been involved in excess of five years (*Table 1*). Females reported modestly longer periods of use than males, median 4.80 and 4.00 years for females and males, respectively.

Abstinence of moderate duration was common among these relatively young heroin users. Eighty-one percent of male users and a somewhat smaller proportion, 65 percent, of female users met our definition of abstention for at least a year prior to reinterview. A majority of the abstainers had remained heroin free for three or more years (*Table 2*).

A sizable proportion of users in the sample reported regular frequency of heroin use at levels suggesting nonaddicted or controlled use. Just about half were daily users, while a quarter of the males and 13 percent of the females used only a few times a month or even less often (*Table 3*). Of interest, frequency of use was only moderately correlated with length of use. More frequent users tended to have used for longer periods of time; nonetheless, 31 percent of casual users (few

Table 1

Length of Heroin Careers by Ages 18-23

	MALE (N=43)	FEMALE (N=26)
Less than 1 year	16%	13%
1 to 2 years	20	13
2 to 3 years	10	13
3 to 5 years	25	29
5 years or more	29	33
Median years used	4.0	4.8

Table 2

Time Since Last Heroin Use: Abstainers only

(from time of second interview)

	MALES (35)	FEMALES (17)
1, up to 2 years ago	15%	10%
2, up to 3 years ago	28	-
3, up to 4 years ago	25	33
4, up to 5 years ago	10	57
5, up to 6 years ago	10	-
6, up to 7 years ago	7	-
8, up to 9 years ago	5	-

Table 3

Frequency of Heroin Use

	MALES (43)	FEMALES (26)
Every day	47%	58%
Few times per week	29	29
Few times per month	10	13
Once a month	4	-
Few times a year	10	-

times a month or less) continued using for at least three years (*Table 4*).

The majority of heroin users had entered treatment at some point during their careers: half of the males (21 of 43) and 62 percent of the females (16 of 26) entered a treatment program at least once between 1969 and 1976. Not unexpectedly, relapse after first-time treatment was widespread. Only about half the individuals entering treatment reported that they last used heroin in the same year that they first entered treatment (*Table 5*). The length of heroin use *after* first treatment entry was normally less than three years, a finding no doubt influenced by the timing of data collection, but a few individuals continued to use heroin for as long as seven years after reported date of first entering treatment. Although the probability of entering treatment increased with more frequent use, treatment experience was reported by even some of the more casual users (*Table 6*).

Annual Hazard Probabilities

Analysis of annual probabilities of abstinence provided results which were consistent with data regarding cumulative lengths of heroin use reported above. Males' annual absti-

Table 4

Length of Heroin Use Careers by Frequency of Use

	Every day (35)	Few times per week (20)	Few times per month or less (14)
0, up to 1 year	10%	13%	12%
1, up to 2 years	12	5	38
2, up to 3 years	3	21	19
3, up to 4 years	22	13	7
4, up to 5 years	14	13	-
5, up to 6 years	12	9	18
6 years and more	27	26	6

Table 5

Post Treatment Heroin Careers*

(duration of use after treatment entry)

	MALES (19)	FEMALES (15)
Last used in same year as entered treatment	45%**	53%**
Last used 1, up to 2 years after entry	9	37
Last used 2, up to 3 years after entry	23	-
Last used 3, up to 4 years after entry	9	5
Last used 4, up to 5 years after entry	-	-
Last used 5, up to 6 years after entry	5	5
Last used 6, up to 7 years after entry	-	-
Last used 7, up to 8 years after entry	9	-

* Base population are all those who ever entered treatment, regardless of whether currently using or abstaining.

** Two women and one man entered treatment in year of interview.

Table 6

Treatment Entry by Frequency of Heroin Use

	% Treated
Every day (35)	63%
Few times per week (20)	48%
Few times per month or less (14)	37%

nence rates exceeded females' more often than the reverse but differences fell within the limits of normal sampling error (*Table 7*). For example, 12% of the 43 male heroin users abstained in the first year of use compared to 7% of female

Table 7

Annual Hazard Probabilities of Abstaining from Heroin Use*

Length of Use (Years)	MALES		FEMALES	
	Heroin Users	Hazard Prob.	Heroin Users	Hazard Prob.
Less than 1	43	.12	26	.07
1, up to 2	38	.21	24	.08
2, up to 3	29	.12	22	.18
3, up to 4	25	.31	18	.17
4, up to 5	17	.20	15	.20
5, up to 6	13	.13	12	.17
6, up to 7	9	.37	7	.14
7, up to 8	5	-	5	.20
8, up to 9	2	-	3	-
9, up to 10	1	1.00	-	-

* Maximum likelihood estimates of simple hazard model, with gender as single independent variable produced insignificant coefficient .216, S.E. .325, p=.51. Kolmogorov-Smirnov Two-Sample Test confirmed these results.

users. Of the remaining heroin users, 21% of the 38 males at risk, compared to 8% of the 24 female heroin users at risk, achieved abstinence in their second year of use. (Note that the hazard probability is a rate or percent of those still at risk, which is the total pool of users minus those who have already achieved abstinence.)

Event-History Analysis

Despite the rough parity in annual abstinence, analysis of the event-history model revealed marked differences between young black men and women in the role of treatment in effecting abstinence (*Table 8*). The first finding of note is that the interaction term for gender and treatment was significant (b = −1.780, p < .05). This signifies that treatment had a different effect on male and female abstinence rates. In the presence of the interaction term, the highly significant main treatment effect (b = 1.898, p < .005) indicates that among women treatment made a large difference in annual abstinence rates. The significant gender variable indicates that without treatment, males had higher abstinence rates than females (b = 1.293, p < .05). These results are now discussed in greater detail.

Female heroin users' rates of abstinence increased dramatically following first-time treatment entry. After adjusting for gender differences in age, frequency, and duration of heroin use, in each year following treatment entry the odds that a woman heroin user would abstain increased more than six times (exp.(1.898) = 6.672) over what they were for an untreated woman. Treatment intervention was clearly an essential factor in reducing the length of young black females' heroin careers.

Turning to males, the impact of treatment on the length of their heroin careers was far less substantial. The effect of treatment for males (obtained by adding the main treatment coefficient to the interaction term (1.898 − 1.780 = .118) was positive but of trivial magnitude. This indicates that the rates of abstinence which young black males achieved through treatment were but marginally greater than those arrived at naturally without treatment.

Among the control variables which were tested, only age proved to have a significant impact on rates of abstinence. Older users abstained at higher rates than younger users. Neither the frequency of heroin use nor the length of time used materially influenced the likelihood of annual abstinence independently of the other variables which were tested.[c]

In short, while neither tabular analysis nor the hazard probabilities model showed a significant difference between the length of men and women's heroin careers, the more elaborated event-history model demonstrated significant gender differences in the pathways to abstinence. To a much greater extent than males, young black females relied on therapeutic intervention to achieve abstinence.

Table 8

Event-History Analysis:

Annual Rates of Abstaining from Heroin Use

(standard errors in parentheses)

Variables	b
Sex	1.293*
	(.505)
Post Treatment Effect	1.898***
	(.576)
Sex x Treatment	-1.780*
	(.714)
Current Age	.501***
	(.174)
Frequency of Use	.104
	(.169)
Duration of Use	-.117
	(.109)

Period Specific Abstaining Effects (contrasted with 1969)

	1970	-.365
		(.965)
	1971	.906
		(.851)
	1972	.527
		(.906)

Table 8 (cont.)

1973	.810
	(.958)
1974	-.786
	(1.162)
1975	-.162
	(1.184)
Model Chi-square#	21.75***
d.f.	6

*p < .05   **p < .01   ***p < .005

Model Chi-square measures improvement in fit due to explanatory

variables net of period specific effects.

SUMMARY AND DISCUSSION

The study reported here is part of a broader program of longitudinal research which has two objectives. The first is to examine antecedents, correlates and consequences of non-medical substance use. The second is to probe gender distinct meanings in these patterns of drug use and treatment experience. By analyzing these experiences in an inner city black population who are at high risk of drug involvement and its sequelae, findings from this investigation are intended to complement those from the predominantly white samples upon which the major part of research into drug use and treatment behavior have thus far been based.

A majority of both male (81% of 43) and female (65% of 26) nonexperimental heroin users in this sample had discontinued heroin use for at least one year prior to reinterview (at ages 18–23). They have been termed "abstainers" in this study. The gender difference in overall abstention rates was not large enough to indicate a statistically true difference between males and females. In addition, approximately half of the nonexperimental heroin users in the sample (49% of males, 62% of females) had undergone at least one treatment episode. Here again, the gender specific rates identified a difference which might have arisen by chance. On the basis of dates of heroin use and of treatment which respondents reported, in approximately half the cases heroin use continued after entering treatment (55% of treated males and 47% of females).

An earlier analysis of these data was focused on gender differences in the timing of treatment entry[24] and showed that males entered treatment earlier in their heroin careers than females did. The observed female pattern of delayed treatment entry held even after controlling for male and female differences in age and heaviness of use.

Research reported in the present paper extends the analysis of gender differences in drug use and treatment experiences to an examination of the role of treatment in achieving abstinence from heroin. Applying event-history methodology, annual rates of abstinence following first treatment entry were compared to those occurring spontaneously, i.e., without treatment, controlling for differences in age and in frequency and duration of heroin use.

The simple hazard probability analysis of annual abstinence rates confirmed the earlier tabular findings that males and females did not differ significantly in their cumulative probabilities of abstinence. The more elaborated event-history model demonstrated, however, that treatment played a significantly different role in men's and women's achieving abstinence.

The benefits of treatment were much more evident for females than males. For each year of use prior to entering treatment, a woman's probability of abstinence was much lower than a man's. But after entering treatment, the annual probability that a woman would abstain from heroin use was not only greatly enhanced relative to what it was without treatment, it was also somewhat greater than the post-treatment probability for a man. As for men, the probability of abstaining in any given year increased only marginally after treatment entry. This finding obtained with gender differences in patterns of use such as frequency and duration and the age of the user taken into account.

As to the independent effects of the control variables, the only one which influenced the probability of abstinence in any given year was age: older users (i.e., up to age 23) were more likely to have discontinued use regardless of duration or frequency of use.

The primary finding that males had almost equal likelihood of abstinence with and without treatment is not intended to convey that treatment is inefficacious for males. The general proposition that some people need treatment to abstain while others can abstain without it seems a proper one. One may logically infer that individuals who entered treatment found it more difficult to stop using heroin than those who did not. Hence even if treated rates of abstinence among males only equaled those achieved naturally, the rate for the treated individuals might still reflect a higher rate than would have prevailed had those males who entered treatment not done so. We do not claim to have evidence that treated and nontreated users were "randomly" drawn from the same heroin user population, but it should be emphasized that the nearly equal rates of treated and natural abstinence observed for men were determined *after netting out* differences in age, frequency and duration of use. Therefore, we can at least rule out these three variables as possible suppressors.

The finding that treatment appears to play a much more crucial role in ending females' use than males' adds to the picture of gender specific patterns in drug use behavior which has been emerging in this research: females, if less likely to experiment with heroin in the first place, were more prone to deeper involvement once begun (suggested by their average greater frequency and longer term of use).[6,20] It was also borne out in female heroin users' greater distinction from other young women (e.g., higher fertility, school dropout, and reported rates of "hustling" as a source of income) when compared to the relative standing of male heroin users vis à vis other young black men in the sample. In an earlier study of timing of first treatment entry up to age 23 (mentioned above) males were observed to enter treatment at a relatively constant rate during their heroin using period while females' entry clustered after three years of use. Although females in the sample, for as yet undetermined reasons, tended to enter treatment after longer periods of use than males, the present study shows that they nonetheless relied more heavily on it as a pathway to abstinence. Unfortunately, numbers of treated cases did not permit separate analysis by treatment modality. We do know that females' average treatment episodes were longer than males' as was their cumulative length of time in treatment across all reported episodes.[d] Equivalent proportions of young treated males and females in this study had been in residential treatment (about a third). Six in ten females reported a methadone clinic while males were more dispersed between that modality (23%) and hospital (19%), prison (13%) and military units (6%). These differences reflect real differences in the life styles and life situations of black male and female youth.

It is interesting to conceptualize these gender differences in treatment behavior and in abstinence as contingent upon available psychosocial supports, i.e., internal and external, needed for spontaneous abstinence from heroin use. Here we are thinking about likely differences in interpersonal networks, in social role alternatives, in introjected norms as well as other socially patterned experiences which impact on coping resources, skills and social expectancies. We hypothesize, for example, that interpersonal networks are more tolerant of black male heroin use than female. These imputed gender differences will be tested more fully in the third round of this study which is currently underway.

When analysis centers on comparison of treated and untreated users, entry into treatment clearly represents a choice point: a problematic juncture in a heroin career. Treatment intervention is but one variable component in a longer sequence of events describing alternative pathways out of heroin use. Not all heroin users enter treatment to kick their habit. Those who do, enter at varying stages in their heroin careers. They may experience numerous treatment episodes during the course of drug use.[41] When viewed as part of a natural history of heroin use, treatment entry—whether self or externally imposed—represents an opportunity for individuals to acquire resources and skills needed for ending drug dependency. For those among whom drug use does not cease without treatment, their entry into treatment *ipso facto* signifies that the resources and supports needed for abstinence were lacking in their natural environment.

Conceptualized in these terms, treatment becomes an issue of behavior change and of the imparting and acquisition of skills and resources needed to overcome inadequate interpersonal and role supports. Heroin treatment is not unlike other programs for behavior change. Hunt et al.[42] report that smoking cessation and alcohol programs succeed only 25 percent of the time in producing behavior change sustained for at least one year. Given the magnitude of the task, it may be inappropriate to judge the success of treatment on the basis of any single episode. Instead, treatment intervention might better be viewed as a possible sequence of exposures of varying lengths, depending on what different individuals require. It is this approach which we will elaborate in later stages of this research program.

NOTES

a. In compliance with requests of the study's Community Advisory Committee, no direct questions about drug use were included in the first interviews in adolescence. To estimate the consistency and accuracy of drug histories, age at onset of heroin use reported on second interview was compared with information available for eight members of the group who had been ascertained (through unsolicited self report, and/or parent, physician or interviewer report) to have been using heroin at time of first interview. In no case was the retrospective report of first use inconsistent with the coterminous report at time of first interview. Other researchers' have consistently reported satisfactory reliability in self reports of illicit drug use.[3,9,11,34-39] The conclusion of these investigators is that, when there is bias, it tends toward underreport not to overreport or non report and to understate current, rather than earlier use.

b. For current users reinterviewed in 1975, year of last use was 1974.

c. When tested for gender interaction, frequency and/or duration still had no effect. It is possible that these negative findings resulted from specification error. However, no significant findings appeared when the variables were changed from interval measures into dichotomies.

d. Length of treatment episodes, individually and cumulatively, was calculated for 13 of 21 treated males and 14 of 16 treated females. Missing cases represent those who provided only year of treatment, not month and are clustered more heavily among males and especially those males who reported detox as their modality.

| | *Male* | | *Female* | |
	$\bar{X}$	(S.D.)	$\bar{X}$	(S.D.)
Months per treatment episode	9.4	(13.4)	10.2	(10.5)
Cumulative months in treatment	11.0	(13.5)	14..1	(13.4)

REFERENCES

1. Johnson B. The race, class and irreversibility hypothesis· Myths and research about heroin. In: Rittenhouse JD, ed. The epidemiology of heroin and other narcotics. Rockville, MD: National Institute on Drug Abuse, 1977.

2. Lukoff I. Consequences of use: Heroin and other narcotics. In: Rittenhouse JD ed. The epidemiology of heroin and other narcotics. Rockville, MD: National Institute on Drug Abuse, 1977.

3. Robins LN. Addict Careers. In: Dupont RI, Goldstein A, O'Donnell JA, eds. Handbook on drug abuse. Washington, DC: U.S. Government Printing Office, 1979:325–336.

4. Waldorf D. Natural recovery from opiate addiction: Some social-psychological processes of untreated recovery. J. Drug Issues 1983; 13(2): 237–280.

5. Winick C. The 35 and 40 age dropoff. In: Proceedings of the White House Conference on Narcotic and Drug Abuse. Washington, DC: U.S Government Printing Office, 1962:153–160.

6. Brunswick AF. Black youths and drug-use behavior. In: Beschner GM, Friedman AS, eds. Youth drug abuse. Lexington, MA: Lexington Books, 1979.

7. O'Donnell JA, Voss HL, Clayton R, Slatin G, Room B. Young men and drugs—A nationwide survey. Research Monograph No. 5. Rockville, MD: National Institute on Drug Abuse, 1976.

8. Robins LN. Drug treatment after return in Vietnam veterans. Highlights of the 20th Annual Conference. Perry Point, MD: Veterans Administration, 1975.

9. Robins LN, Murphy GE. Drug use in a normal population of young Negro men. Am. J. Public Health. 1967; 57: 1580–1596.

10. Waldorf D. Biernacki P. Natural recovery from heroin addiction: A review of the incidence literature. J. Drug Issues 1979; 9(2): 281–289.

11. Robins LN. A followup of Vietnam drug users. Special Action Office Monograph Series A, No. 1. Washington, DC: Executive Office of the President, 1973.

12 Robins LN. Estimating addiction rates and locating target populations How decomposition into stages helps. In: Rittenhouse JD ed. The epidemiology of heroin and other narcotics. Rockville, MD: National Institute on Drug Abuse, 1977.

13. Waldorf D. Careers in dope. Englewood Cliffs, NJ: Prentice-Hall, 1973

14. Zinberg NE. Nonaddictive opiate use. In: Dupont RI, Goldstein A, O'Donnell JA, eds. Handbook on drug abuse. Washington, DC: U.S. Government Printing Office, 1979:303–313.

15. Waldorf D. Life without heroin: Some social adjustments during long-term periods of voluntary abstinence Social Problems 1970; 18(2): 228–242.

16. Hunt LG. Prevalence of active heroin use in the United States In: Rittenhouse JD, ed. The epidemiology of heroin and other narcotics. Rockville, MD. National Institute on Drug Abuse, 1977.

17. Bales RN. Outcome research in therapeutic communities for drug abusers: A critical review, 1963–1975. Int. J. Addict. 1979; 14: 1053–1074.

18. Binion VJ. Sex differences in socialization and family dynamics of female and male heroin users. J. Social Issues 1982; 38(2): 77–92.

19. Boyle JM, Brunswick AF. What happened in Harlem? Analysis of a decline in heroin use among a generation unit of urban black youth. J. Drug Issues 1980; 10:109–130.

20. Brunswick AF. Social meanings and developmental needs: Perspectives on black youth's drug abuse. Youth & Society 1980; 11(4): 449–473.

21. Cuskey WB, Wathey RB. Female addiction. Lexington, MA: Lexington Books, 1982.

22. Moise R, Reed BG, Ryan V. Issues in the treatment of heroin addicted women: A comparison of men and women entering two types of drug abuse programs. Int. J. Addict. 1982; 17: 1099–139.

23. Savage LG, Simpson DD. Posttreatment outcome of sex and ethnic groups treated in methadone maintenance, 1969–1972. J. Psychedelic Drugs 1980; 12:55–63.

24. Brunswick AF, Messeri P. Timing of first drug treatment: A longitudinal study of urban black youth. Contemp. Drug Prob., 1985; 2(3): 401–418

25. Tuma NB, Hanna MT, Groeneveld LP. Dynamic analysis of event histories. Am. J. Sociology 1979; 84: 820–854.

26. Brunswick AF, Messeri P. Gender differences in processes of smoking initiation. J. Psychosocial Oncology 1984; 2(1):49–69.

27. Ensminger ME, Brown CH, Kellam SG. Sex differences in antecedents of substance use among adolescents. J. Social Issues 1982; 38: 25–42.

28. Rosenbaum, M. Women on heroin. New Brunswick, NJ: Rutgers University Press, 1981.

29. Sutker PB. Drug dependent women. In: Beschner G, Reed BG, Mondanaro J, eds. Treatment services for drug dependent women, Vol. I. NIDA Treatment Research Monograph Series. Rockville, MD: National Institute on Drug Abuse, 1981:25–51.

30. Tucker MB. Social support and coping: Applications for the study of female drug abuse. J. Social Issues 1982; 38: 117–138.

31. Colten ME. Attitudes, experiences and self-perceptions of heroin addicted mothers. J. Social Issues 1982; 38: 77–92.

32. Brunswick AF. Health consequences of drug use: A longitudinal study of urban black youth. In Mednick SA, Harway, M, Finello KM, eds. Handbook of Longitudinal Research in the U.S., Vol. 2. New York, NY: Praeger Press, 1984: 290–310.

33 Brunswick AF. Health and drug use among black youths: Predictors, concomitants and consequences. Final report to National Institute on Drug Abuse. Grant # ROI-DA-00852. 1980.

34. Ball JC. The reliability and validity of interview data from 59 narcotic drug addicts. Am. J. Soc. 1967; 72(6): 650–654.

35. O'Donnell JA. Survey data as contributors to estimation. In: Rittenhouse JD ed. The epidemiology of heroin and other narcotics. Rockville, MD: National Institute on Drug Abuse, 1977.

36. Robins LN, Davis DH, Nurco DN. How permanent was Vietnam drug addiction? Supplement to Am. J. Public Health 1974; 64: 38–44.

37. Single E, Kandel DB, Johnson BD The reliability and validity of drug use responses in a large scale longitudinal survey. J. Drug Issues 1980; 5(4): 426–443.

38 Stephens R. The truthfulness of addict respondents in research projects. Int. J. Addic. 1972; 7: 549–558.

39 Whitehead PC, Smart RG. Validity and reliability of self reported drug use. Canadian J. Criminology and Corrections 1972; 14: 1–8.

40. Kalbfleisch JD, Prentice RL. The statistical analysis of failure time data. New York, NY: John Wiley and Sons, 1980.

41. National Institute on Drug Abuse (NIDA). Annual data 1981: Data from the client oriented data acquisition process (CODAP), NIDA Statistical Series E, Number 25, 1982.

42. Hunt WA, Matarazzo JD, Weiss SM, Gentry WD. Associative learning, habit, and health behavior. J. Behavior Med. 1979; 2: 111–124

43. Allison P. Discrete time methods for the analysis of event histories. In: Leinhardt S, ed. Sociological methodology. San Francisco, CA: Jossey-Bass Publishers, 1982.

APPENDIX

Analytical Procedure

The hazard is a measure of the underlying propensity of leaving some discrete state (in this case heroin use). If T is a random variable representing the time of leaving a state, then in mathematical notation, the hazard rate of leaving at time t (T = t) is written as (1):

$$\text{Lim} \quad \frac{Pr(t \leqslant T \leqslant t + \Delta t / T > t)}{\Delta t}$$
$$\Delta t \to 0$$

In the present study a discrete time representation of the hazard was calculated on an annual basis (Δt = a year).[43] Specifically, it was the probability that an individual using heroin through the start of year t($Pr\ T > t$) will cease use by the end of that year ($Pr(t < T \leqslant t + \Delta t)$).

The event-history model specifies the hazard probability measuring the risk of abstinence (leaving the state of heroin use) as a joint function of several variable attributes of sample members. The independent variables of the event-history model test for differing conditions that are hypothesized to give rise to variations in the hazard probability across individuals.

Several functional forms for relating the hazard to a set of explanatory variables have been proposed. Here we adopted a linear logistic formulation (2):

$$R_i(t) = \frac{\exp(A(t) + B_1 Z_{i1}(t) + B_2 Z_{12}(t) + \ldots + B_n Z_{in}(t)}{1 + \exp(A(t) + B_1 Z_{i1}(t) + B_2 Z_{i2}(t) + \ldots + B_2 Z_{in}(t)}$$

or

$$\ln[R_i(t)/(1 - R_i(t)] = A(t) + B_1 Z_{i1}(t) + B_2 Z_{i2}(t) + \ldots + B_n Z_{in}(t)$$

$R_i(t)$ is the hazard probability for individual i in time period t, with time-varying attributes $Z_{i1}(t)$ through $Z_{in}(t)$. The B's in the equation measure variation in hazard rates due to covariates Z_1 through Z_n.

"A(t)" measures longitudinal changes in the hazard probability which are assumed to influence uniformly all sample members. The functional form of A(t) can be arbitrarily specified. For the present study A(t) is specified as a step function, adjusting for unspecified exogenous changes in historical conditions which may introduce inter-year variation in the sample's baseline hazard probability. (A baseline hazard is the probability of abstinence for an individual with zero values on all independent variables, $Z = 0$).

SELECTIVE GUIDE TO CURRENT REFERENCE SOURCES ON TOPICS DISCUSSED IN THIS ISSUE

Alcohol and Substance Use and Abuse in Women and Children

Lynn Kasner Morgan, MLS
James E. Raper, Jr., MSLS

Each issue of *Advances in Alcohol & Substance Abuse* features a section offering suggestions on where to look for further information on topics discussed in that issue. In this issue, our intent is to guide readers to selected sources of current information on alcohol and substance use and abuse in women and children.

Some reference sources utilize designated terminology (controlled vocabularies) which must be used to find material on topics of interest. For these we shall indicate a sample of available search terms so that the reader can access suitable sources for his/her purposes. Other reference tools use keywords or free-text terms (generally from the title of the docu-

The authors are affiliated with the Gustave L. and Janet W. Levy Library, The Mount Sinai Medical Center of New York, Inc., One Gustave L. Levy Place, New York, NY 10029.

137

ment or the name of the agency or conference listed). In searching the latter, the user should also look under synonyms for the concept in question.

An asterisk (*) appearing before a published source indicates that all or part of that source is in machine-readable form and can be accessed through an online data base search. Data base searching is recommended for retrieving sources of information that coordinates multiple concepts or subject areas. A data base search on this topic will be especially useful since the search may be limited by sex and age variables. This is not possible when using the printed indexes.

Readers are encouraged to consult their librarians for further assistance before undertaking research on a topic.

Suggestions regarding the content and organization of this section are welcome.

1. INDEXING AND ABSTRACTING SOURCES

Place of publication, publisher, start date, and frequency of publication are noted.

Biological Abstracts and *Biological Abstracts/RRM*. Philadelphia, BioSciences Information Service, 1926– , semimonthly.
    See: Abstracts and content summaries in pharmacology, psychiatry, toxicology sections.
    See: Keyword-in-context subject index.
Chemical Abstracts. Columbus, Ohio, American Chemical Society, 1907– , weekly.
    See: *Index Guide* for cross-referencing and indexing policies.
    See: *General Subject Index* terms, such as drug dependence, drug-drug interactions.
    See: Keyword subject indexes.
Dissertation Abstracts International. Section B. The Sciences and Engineering. Ann Arbor, Mich., University Microfilms, 1969– , monthly (continues *Microfilm Abstracts* and *Dissertation Abstracts*, 1938–1968).
    See: Keyword-in-context subject index.
Excerpta Medica: Clinical Biochemistry. Section 29. Amster-

dam, The Netherlands, Excerpta Medica, v.27, 1973– , 32 issues per year.
See: Subject index.
Excerpta Medica: Drug Dependence. Section 40. Amsterdam, The Netherlands, Excerpta Medica, v.8, 1980– , 6 issues per year.
See: Subject index.
Excerpta Medica: Internal Medicine. Section 6. Amsterdam, The Netherlands, Excerpta Medica, 1947– , 30 issues per year.
See: Subject index.
Excerpta Medica: Obstetrics and Gynecology. Section 10. Amsterdam, The Netherlands, Excerpta Medica, 1948– , 20 issues per year.
See: Subject index.
Excerpta Medica: Pediatrics and Pediatric Surgery. Section 7. Amsterdam, The Netherlands, Excerpta Medica, v.26, 1972–, 20 issues per year.
See: Subject index.
Excerpta Medica: Pharmacology. Section 30. Amsterdam, The Netherlands, Excerpta Medica, v.57, 1983– , 20 issues per year.
See: Alcoholism, drug addiction sections.
See: Subject index.
Excerpta Medica: Psychiatry. Section 32. Amsterdam, The Netherlands, Excerpta Medica, v.22, 1969– , 20 issues per year.
See: Addiction, alcoholism sections.
See: Subject index.
Excerpta Medica: Public Health, Social Medicine and Hygiene. Section 17. Amsterdam, The Netherlands, Excerpta Medica, 1955– , 20 issues per year.
See: Addiction, drug control sections.
See: Subject index.
Excerpta Medica: Rehabilitation and Physical Medicine. Section 19. Amsterdam, The Netherlands, Excerpta Medica, v.7, 1964– , 10 issues per year.
See: Subject index.
Excerpta Medica: Toxicology. Section 52. Amsterdam, The Netherlands, Excerpta Medica, 1983– , 20 issues per year.
See: Subject index.
Index Medicus. (including *Bibliography of Medical Reviews*).

Bethesda, Md., National Library of Medicine, 1960– , monthly.

See: *MeSH* terms, such as adolescence, alcohol drinking, alcoholic intoxication, alcoholism, cannabis, cannabis abuse, child, cocaine, drug interactions, fetal alcohol syndrome, maternal-fetal exchange, parent-child relations, substance abuse, substance dependence, substance use disorders, women.

Index to Scientific Reviews. Philadelphia, Institute for Scientific Information, 1974– , semiannual.

See: Permuterm keyword subject index.

See: Citation index.

International Pharmaceutical Abstracts. Washington, D.C., American Society of Hospital Pharmacists, 1964– , semimonthly.

See: IPA subject terms, such as alcoholism, cannabis, cocaine, drug abuse, toxicity.

Psychological Abstracts. Washington, D.C., American Psychological Association, 1927– , monthly.

See: Index terms, such as addiction, alcohol drinking attitudes, alcohol rehabilitation, alcoholism, cocaine, drug abuse, drug addiction, drug rehabilitation, heroin addiction, marijuana usage, social drinking.

Public Affairs Information Service Bulletin. New York, Public Affairs Information Service, 1915– , semimonthly.

See: PAIS subject headings, such as alcohol-and-youth, drugs-and-youth, women-drug-problem, women-liquor-problem, youth-liquor-problem.

Science Citation Index. Philadelphia, Institute for Scientific Information, 1961– , bimonthly.

See: Permuterm keyword subject index.

See: Citation index.

Social Sciences Citation Index. Philadelphia, Institute for Scientific Information, 1973– , 3 issues per year.

See: Permuterm keyword subject index.

See: Citation index.

Social Work Research and Abstracts. New York, National Association of Social Workers, 1965– , quarterly.

See: Fields of service sections, such as alcoholism and drug addiction.

See: Subject index.

Sociological Abstracts. San Diego, Calif., International Sociological Association, 1953– , 5 issues per year.
See: Subject index terms, such as addict/addicts/addicted/ addictive/addiction, alcohol, alcoholic/alcoholics/alcoholism, drinking/drinkers, drug/drugs, drug addict/drug addicts/ drug addiction, heroin, marijuana.

2. CURRENT AWARENESS PUBLICATIONS

Current Contents: Clinical Practice. Philadelphia, Institute for Scientific Information, 1973– , weekly.
See: Keyword index.
Current Contents: Life Sciences. Philadelphia, Institute for Scientific Information, 1958– , weekly.
See: Keyword index.
Current Contents: Social and Behavioral Sciences. Philadelphia, Institute for Scientific Information, 1969– , weekly.
See: Keyword index.

3. BOOKS

Andrews, Theodora. *A Bibliography of Drug Abuse, Including Alcohol and Tobacco.* Littleton, Colo., Libraries Unlimited, 1977.
Andrews, Theodora. *A Bibliography of Drug Abuse. Supplement 1977–1980.* Littleton, Colo., Libraries Unlimited, 1981.
Medical Books and Serials in Print: An Index to Literature in the Health Sciences. New York, R. R. Bowker Co., annual.
See: Library of Congress subject headings, such as alcohol, alcoholics, alcoholism, cocaine, drug abuse, hallucinogenic drugs, heroin habit, liquor problem, marihuana, narcotic habit, stimulants, women.
National Library of Medicine Current Catalog. Bethesda, Md., National Library of Medicine, 1966– , quarterly.
See: *MeSH* terms as noted in Section 1 under *Index Medicus.*

4. U. S. GOVERNMENT PUBLICATIONS

Monthly Catalog of United States Government Publications. Washington, D.C., U.S. Government Printing Office, 1895–, monthly.

    See: Following agencies: Alcohol, Drug Abuse and Mental Health Administration, National Institute of Mental Health, National Institute on Drug Abuse.

    See: Subject headings, derived chiefly from the Library of Congress, such as alcohol, alcoholism, children, cocaine, drug abuse, drug habit, hallucinogenic drugs, liquor problem, marihuana, narcotic habit, stimulants, women, youth.

    See: Keyword title index.

5. ONLINE BIBLIOGRAPHIC DATA BASES

Only those data bases which have no single print equivalent are included in this section. Print sources which have online data base equivalents are noted throughout this guide by the asterisk (*) which appears before the title. If you do not have direct access to these data bases, consult a librarian who is a computer search analyst for assistance.

DRUG INFO/ALCOHOL USE/ABUSE (Hazelden Foundation, Center City, Minn., and Drug Information Service Center, College of Pharmacy, University of Minnesota, Minneapolis Minn.).

    Use: Subject headings, such as addiction, adolescent, alcohol, alcoholism, cannabis, children, cocaine, drinking pattern, drug abuse, drug dependence, drug use, drug use pattern, heroin, marihuana.

    Use: Keywords.

FAMILY RESOURCES DATABASE (National Council on Family Relations and Inventory of Marriage and Family Literature Project, Minneapolis, Minn.).

    Use: Classification codes, such as 018W (working mothers), 041 (women's issues), 090D (drug abuse), 096 (families with alcoholics), 111A (adolescence).

    Use: keywords.

MAGAZINE INDEX (Information Access Co., Belmont, Calif.).
    Use: Keywords.
MENTAL HEALTH ABSTRACTS (IFI/Plenum Data Co., Alexandria, Va.).
    Use: Keywords.
NATIONAL NEWSPAPER INDEX (Information Access Co., Belmont, Calif.).
    Use: Keywords.
NTIS (National Technical Information Service, U.S. Dept. of Commerce, Springfield, Va.).
    Use: Keywords.
PRE-MED (BRS Bibliographic Retrieval Services, Inc., Latham, New York).
    Use: Keywords.
PSYCALERT (American Psychological Association, Washington, D.C.).
    Use: Keywords.

6. HANDBOOKS, DIRECTORIES, GRANT SOURCES, ETC.

Annual Register of Grant Support. Chicago, Marquis Academic Media/Marquis Who's Who, annual.
    See: Children and youth; medicine; pediatrics; pharmacology; psychiatry, psychology, mental health; women sections.
Encyclopedia of Associations. 20th ed. Detroit, Gale Research Co., 1986, c1985. (occasional supplements between editions).
    See: Subject index.
*Foundation Directory. New York, The Foundation Center, biennial (updated between editions by *Foundation Directory Supplement*).
    See: Index of foundations.
    See: Index of foundations by state and city.
    See: Index of donors, trustees, and administrators.
    See: Index of fields of interest.
Research Awards Index. Bethesda, Md., National Institutes of Health, Division of Research Grants, annual.
    See: Drug abuse terms in the index volume.

7. JOURNAL LISTINGS

Ulrich's International Periodicals Directory. 24th ed. New
York, R. R. Bowker Co., 1985, (updated between editions
by *Ulrich's Quarterly*).
> See: Subject categories, such as children and youth,
> drug abuse and alcoholism, women's interests.

8. AUDIOVISUAL PROGRAMS

The Health Sciences Videolog. New York, Video Forum, 1981.
> See: Subject index terms, such as alcoholism, drug
> abuse, drug dependence.

National Library of Medicine Audiovisuals Catalog. Bethesda, Md., National Library of Medicine, 1979– , annual.
> See: *MeSH* terms as noted in Section 1 under *Index
> Medicus.*

9. GUIDES TO UPCOMING MEETINGS

Scientific Meetings. San Diego, Calif., Scientific Meetings
Publications, quarterly.
> See: Subject indexes.
> See: Association listing.

World Meetings: Medicine. New York, Macmillan Pub. Co.,
quarterly.
> See: Keyword index.
> See: Sponsor directory and index.

10. PROCEEDINGS OF MEETINGS

Conference Papers Index. Louisville, Ky., Data Courier,
1973–, monthly.

Directory of Published Proceedings. White Plains, N.Y., In-
terDok Corp., 1965– , monthly, except July-August, with
annual cumulations.

Index to Scientific and Technical Proceedings. Philadelphia,

Institute for Scientific Information, 1978– , monthly with semiannual cumulations.

11. SPECIALIZED RESEARCH CENTERS

Research Centers Directory. 10th ed. Detroit, Gale Research Co., 1985–86, c1985 (updated by *New Research Centers*).

12. SPECIAL LIBRARY COLLECTIONS

Ash, L., comp. *Subject Collections*. 5th ed. New York, R. R. Bowker Co., 1978.
Directory of Special Libraries and Information Centers. 9th ed. Detroit, Gale Research Co., 1985 (updates by *New Special Libraries*).

Information for Authors

Advances in Alcohol & Substance Abuse publishes original articles and topical review articles related to all areas of substance abuse. Each publication will be issue-oriented and may contain both basic science and clinical papers.

All submitted manuscripts are read by the editors. Many manuscripts may be further reviewed by consultants. Comments from reviewers will be returned with the rejected manuscripts when it is believed that this may be helpful to the author(s).

The content of *Advances in Alcohol & Substance Abuse* is protected by copyright. Manuscripts are accepted for consideration with the understanding that their contents, all or in part, have not been published elsewhere and will not be published elsewhere except in abstract form or with the express consent of the editor. Author(s) of accepted manuscripts will receive a form to sign for transfer of author's(s') copyright.

The editor reserves the right to make those revisions necessary to achieve maximum clarity and conciseness as well as uniformity to style. *Advances in Alcohol & Substance Abuse* accepts no responsibility for statements made by contributing author(s).

MANUSCRIPT PREPARATION

A double-spaced original and two copies (including references, legends, and footnotes) should be submitted. The manuscript should have margins of at least 4 cm, with subheadings used at appropriate intervals to aid in presentation. There is no definite limitation on length, although a range of fifteen to twenty typed pages is desired.

A cover letter should accompany the manuscript containing the name, address, and phone number of the individual who will be specifically responsible for correspondence.

Title Page

The first page should include title, subtitle (if any), first name, and last name of each author, with the highest academic degree obtained. Each author's academic and program affiliation(s) should be noted, including the name of the department(s) and institution(s) to which the work should be attributed; disclaimers (if any); and the name and address of the author to whom reprint requests should be addressed. Any acknowledgements of financial support should also be listed.

Abstracts

The second page should contain an abstract of not more than 150 words.

References

References should be typed double space on separate pages and arranged according to their order in the text. In the text the references should be in superscript arabic numerals. The form of references should conform to the Index Medicus (National Library of Medicine) style. Sample references are illustrated below:

1. Brown MJ, Salmon D, Rendell M. Clonidine hallucinations. Ann Intern Med. 1980; 93:456-7.
2. Friedman HJ, Lester D. A critical review of progress towards an animal model of alcoholism. In: Blum K, ed. Alcohol and opiates: neurochemical and behavioral mechanisms. New York: Academic Press, 1977:1-19.
3. Berne E. Principles of group treatment. New York: Oxford University Press, 1966.

Reference to articles in press must state name of journal and, if possible, volume and year. References to unpublished material should be so indicated in parentheses in the text.

It is the responsibility of the author(s) to check references against the original source for accuracy both in manuscript and in galley proofs.

Tables and Figures

Tables and figures should be unquestionably clear so that their meaning is understandable without the text. Tables should be typed double space on separate sheets with number and title. Symbols for units should be confined to column headings. Internal, horizontal, and vertical lines may be omitted. The following footnote symbols should be used:* † ‡ § ¶

Figures should be submitted as glossy print photos, untrimmed and unmounted. The label pasted on the back of each illustration should contain the name(s) of author(s) and figure number, with top of figure being so indicated. Photomicrographs should have internal scale markers, with the original magnification as well as stain being used noted. If figures are of patients, the identities should be masked or a copy of permission for publication included. If the figure has been previously published, permission must be obtained from the previous author(s) and copyright holder(s). Color illustrations cannot be published.

Manuscripts and other communications should be addressed to:

Barry Stimmel, MD
Mount Sinai School of Medicine
One Gustave L. Levy Place
Annenberg 5-12
New York, New York 10029

T - #0040 - 160425 - C0 - 229/152/9 [11] - CB - 9780866565752 - Gloss Lamination